Fertile Bonds

UNIVERSITY PRESS OF FLORIDA

Florida A&M University, Tallahassee
Florida Atlantic University, Boca Raton
Florida Gulf Coast University, Ft. Myers
Florida International University, Miami
Florida State University, Tallahassee
New College of Florida, Sarasota
University of Central Florida, Orlando
University of Florida, Gainesville
University of North Florida, Jacksonville
University of South Florida, Tampa
University of West Florida, Pensacola

Fertile Bonds

Bedouin Class, Kinship, and Gender
in the Bekaa Valley

Suzanne E. Joseph

UNIVERSITY PRESS OF FLORIDA

Gainesville / Tallahassee / Tampa / Boca Raton

Pensacola / Orlando / Miami / Jacksonville / Ft. Myers / Sarasota

The publication of this book was made possible in part by a grant from the College of Arts and Sciences at Zayed University, United Arab Emirates.

This book may be available in an electronic edition.

22 21 20 19 18 17   6 5 4 3 2 1

First cloth printing, 2013
First paperback printing, 2017

Library of Congress Cataloging-in-Publication Data
Joseph, Suzanne E.
Fertile bonds : Bedouin class, kinship, and gender in the Bekaa Valley / Suzanne E. Joseph.
p. cm.
Includes bibliographical references and index.
ISBN 978-0-8130-4461-3 (cloth: alk. paper)
ISBN 978-0-8130-5410-0 (pbk.)
1. Bedouins—Lebanon—Biqa' Valley. 2. Families—Lebanon—Biqa' Valley. 3. Fertility, Human—Lebanon—Biqa' Valley. 4. Sex role—Lebanon—Biqa' Valley. 5. Biqa' Valley (Lebanon)—Social life and customs. I. Title.
DS80.55.B43J67 2013
304.6089'927205692—dc23   2013007074

The University Press of Florida is the scholarly publishing agency for the State University System of Florida, comprising Florida A&M University, Florida Atlantic University, Florida Gulf Coast University, Florida International University, Florida State University, New College of Florida, University of Central Florida, University of Florida, University of North Florida, University of South Florida, and University of West Florida.

University Press of Florida
15 Northwest 15th Street
Gainesville, FL 32611-2079
http://www.upf.com

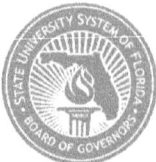

Contents

List of Figures   vi
List of Tables   vii
Acknowledgments   ix
Note on Transliteration   xi

1. Introduction and Overview   1
2. Nomadic Lives in Transition   23
3. (Un)Stratified Reproduction: Class, Tribe, and Culture   42
4. Gender Myths and Demographic Realities   73
5. Marriage between Kin   95
6. Population and Poverty: A Capitalist Trap?   117
7. Class Differentiation of Demographic Regimes   133
8. Demography on the Nomadic Periphery   154
9. Conclusions   173

Notes   181
Bibliography   205
Index   225

Figures

2.1. Bedouin women's parental occupation   31

3.1. Bedouin woman with forearm and facial tattoos   44

3.2. Syrian Bedouin woman welcoming visitors to her family's tent house   47

3.3. Bedouin tribal shaykh serving coffee to welcome guest (author)   48

3.4. Bedouin woman roping and milking sheep as her daughter watches   59

3.5. Bedouin pastoral household in their spring tent   61

Tables

2.1. Observed and weighted completed family size distributions of the mothers of informants by birth cohort 34

2.2. Completed family sizes of 102 postreproductive Bedouin women born 1942–1960 35

2.3. Comparison of Bedouin period and cohort fertility 36

3.1. Household ownership status of sheep/goats, cows, and land, 2000–2001 50

3.2. Size of land holdings among households that own land, 2000–2001 51

3.3. Household herd size of sheep/goats among households that own herds, 2000–2001 52

3.4. Distribution of cows among households that own cows, 2000–2001 52

3.5. Household ownership status of the means of production by occupation, 2000–2001 62

3.6. Mean number of live births and survivors by occupation among 102 postreproductive Bedouin women 63

4.1. Mortality measures on ever born female children of 240 Bedouin women 80

4.2. Mortality measures on ever born male children of 240 Bedouin women 80

4.3. Mean number of live births by polygynous status among 102 postreproductive Bedouin women 88

5.1. Prevalence of Bedouin consanguineous marriage 96

5.2. Prevalence of Bedouin consanguineous marriage by occupation 110

8.1. The distribution of fertility among seven nomadic societies (classified by five-year age groups) 166

Acknowledgments

This book has been a labor of love in spite of the birth pangs. I am grateful to the following scholars for their comments and suggestions: Charles Peters, Alexandra Brewis Slade, Alan G. Hill, and Lila Abu-Lughod. The author bears sole responsibility for any errors, oversights, or omissions. I would also like to acknowledge the detailed and diligent feedback of an anonymous reviewer solicited by the University Press of Florida. The editor in chief for the press, Amy Gorelick, expressed interest in the book from the very beginning, and for that I am extremely grateful. Cassandra Palmer edited the manuscript with great care and attention to detail. Research for this book was supported by a Boren International Fellowship, an award from the University of Georgia, a Brandeis University Andrew Mellon Fellowship, a travel grant from the University of Massachusetts–Dartmouth, and a new faculty start-up grant from Zayed University. I am deeply grateful to my natal family for their continuous support and encouragement. I must also acknowledge my debt to my former in-laws. Two decades have passed since my first visit to the Bekaa and still our lives continue to intersect and come together—overlapping experiences that are now embodied in the pages of this text. I thank Ahmad Sawwan and his family for their hospitality and kind assistance during my stay in the Bekaa. A special thank-you goes to Nada Raghib and Shaykh Haysam for their unwavering friendship and support. Above all, I wish to express my gratitude to the Bedouin families of the Bekaa Valley who welcomed me into their homes and hearts. Thank you for giving me the kind of experience that, as an anthropologist, you only dream about. I continue to draw inspiration from your histories. For those who do not know the Bedouin, I offer this book, hoping that it does not disappoint my Bedouin hosts.

Note on Transliteration

Most speakers alternated between Lebanese and Bedouin Arabic dialects during conversations with the author. Arabic is transliterated according to the system employed in *The Encyclopaedia of Islam, New Edition*, eds. Peri J. Bearman et al. with some changes: *j* is used instead of *dj*, q instead of ḳ, no underlining of digraphs, and no apostrophe if *alif al-waṣl* is elided (*fī l-bayt* instead of *fī 'l-bayt*; *bī l-dayf* instead of *bī 'l-dayf*). In accordance with convention, the final ending *-iyy* is rendered as *-ī* in *nisbas* such as *Badawī* and for names such as *ʿAlī*. Some personal and place names as well as terms with common English spellings are not transliterated according to this system but left in their anglicized form (e.g., fellah instead of *fallāḥ* and Hauran instead of Ḥawrān).

1

Introduction and Overview

Vital demographic events are at once global and deeply personal. On a personal level, demographic events include if, when, and whom we marry and sometimes divorce; if, when, and how many children we have; and why and when we die. On a global scale, much attention has recently been paid to the demographic divide, or the gulf in birth and death rates among the world's inhabitants. On the one side are poor countries with relatively high fertility rates and low life expectancies. On the other side are wealthy countries with fertility rates so low that population decline and rapid aging are expected. A primary reason for concern over the global demographic divide is not simply the differential pace of population growth but the disparities in human health, economic well-being, and future prosperity implied by these demographic trends.[1] Reducing demographic and health disparities are social-justice issues of concern to social scientists, public-health professionals, policymakers, and the general public.

As a social-justice issue, the demographic divide is believed to contain within itself the seeds of its own problem and apropos solution. Poverty and inequality are frequently depicted as consequences of population growth. Economist and founder of modern demography Thomas Robert Malthus (1766–1834) argued that because of the "natural" imbalance between too many people and too few resources to support them, poverty, misery, and a Hobbesian-like war of all against all are always lurking on the human horizon. The only way to avoid this ill-fated predicament is to delay marriage and reproduction while keeping in check sexual activity prior to marriage. Malthus saw high fertility, which persists in some parts of the global South today, as a negative force that generates pauperism, disease, and death and threatens sustainable economic growth. Malthusianism/neo-Malthusianism continues to shape how we perceive poor peoples and their increase. Modern concerns over population growth can still, in large part, be attributed to racist and classist fears that the Third

World will engulf the North and threaten its power, accelerate outmigration from the South to the North, pollute the environment, and spread disease and criminality.[2]

But the purported dangers of uncontrolled fertility do not end there. High fertility is also believed to be incompatible with the social-justice cause of women's equality and liberation. It is a veritable axiom of social-scientific thought that the historical contraction in family size—both a cause and consequence of the introduction of modern methods of birth control—helped separate sex from reproduction and thus free women "from a chronic round of pregnancy and childbirth."[3] This disentangling of sex from the "exigencies of reproduction" spawned the sexual revolution and is believed to have democratized intimate relations between the genders.[4] While there is no doubt that these changes in reproduction have been revolutionary, we must also probe the underlying misconceptions about women's reproduction in the global South to which they have given rise. Chief among them is the unquestioned assumption that large families are symptomatic of the patriarchal subordination of women.

Bedouin constitute prime examples of Arab-Muslim peoples living on the other side of the population divide with pronounced fertility and population growth rates. Given that the small nuclear family is one of the main hallmarks of modernity and women's liberation, the high fertility of Bedouin women—among the highest fertility levels known to humanity, at over nine children per woman—marks them and others like them situated on the other side of the global demographic divide as a foil to modernity and gender equality. The reproductive-rights and population-control movements have contributed to the pathologization of high fertility, promoting a false dichotomy that equates small families with reproductive freedom, economic well-being, and health advantage and equates large families with reproductive oppression, economic hardship, and health disadvantage. With respect to Arab-Muslim societies, women's subordination and lack of autonomy are believed to be manifested demographically in early and prolific reproduction, polygyny, and close-kin marriages.

The specter of "overpopulation"—attributed to "prolific" reproduction among poor women of color—continues to loom over the social-justice commitment of improving the health and welfare of socially disadvantaged groups. Class and racial polarities of the past have been reproduced in the present. Since its inception, the science of demography has demonstrated interest in social inequality, albeit an often sinister interest in containing poor sectors of bourgeois society in Europe and subjugating racially "inferior" peoples in colonized societies around the world.[5] The aim of the present book is to tell a different story about the demographic lives of women and men living on the poor side of the rich/poor divide.

There is an emerging awareness in the anthropological literature that reproduction cannot be studied in isolation from the political and socioeconomic institutions that define it and are defined by it.[6] As an anthropological demographic study, the present book follows in the wake of previous studies from Europe, Asia, Africa, and Latin America that have examined the role of social class or occupational inequality in shaping microreproductive behavior, and the role of broader political-economic forces in determining the onset and pace of fertility transition.[7] A critical limitation of previous microdemographic research on social-class variation is that much of the historical demographic literature, especially that prior to fertility transition, is confined to western Europe, where there is abundant high-quality parish register data going back centuries. Another limitation is that the demographic experiences of marginal peoples farther removed from consolidated state control, particularly nomadic groups, are seldom incorporated into general insights about social inequality and health. Disciplinary divisions between sociocultural and biological subfields have contributed to the fragmentation of anthropological demographic knowledge, with sociocultural researchers mostly focused on the demography of agrarian village and urban ethnic communities in nation-states, and biological researchers mostly concerned with the demography of "primitives," "preindustrial," or nomadic peoples.[8]

Theoretical divisions are no less apparent. Biodemographers tend to draw on evolutionary theory and human biology (reproductive biology, physiology, and genetics) to understand human demographic behavior, whereas (cultural) anthropological demographers direct attention to the historically and culturally contingent structures of power. The theoretical inclination of anthropological demographers to treat demographic events as products of social action and biodemographers to treat them as products of biological evolution results in a theoretical impasse, leaving the reader without much help in determining the relative merits of each approach. With respect to questions on inequality, such divisions make it difficult to draw broader conclusions about if/how historical processes of class struggle have shaped the demographic experiences of nomadic peoples in peripheral areas of state control. While several ethnographic studies of foraging and pastoral societies suggest an egalitarian sociopolitical order, the issue of how social structure and demography relate to each other remains an open question.

Some scholars have even gone so far as to suggest that egalitarianism, at least in pastoral societies, is a myth.[9]

The present study addresses these questions by analyzing demographic findings from peasant Europe and Asia alongside those from nomadic and seminomadic communities living within and between state boundaries, particularly my own work with Bedouin agropastoralists in the Bekaa Valley, Lebanon.[10] In examining the causes of demographic differentiation, public-health researchers have further pointed out that as socioeconomic conditions improve and the incidence of primarily environmental disease concomitantly declines, biogenetic disorders are going to account for an increasing proportion of worldwide morbidity and mortality.[11] The general assumption is that in societies or social sectors where socioeconomic inequalities are low or have been substantially reduced, biological factors will emerge as the primary determinants of health disparities. A major challenge for demographers and health-oriented researchers is to explore the convergences of biology and politics without naturalizing nurture and socializing nature.

At the core of the book is a comparative ethnographic and demographic study of Bedouin in the Bekaa Valley—one that provides a new basis for understanding the demographic underpinnings of social inequality by considering demographic conjunctures from across the range of egalitarian and class-stratified polities. An anthropological demographic study on the nomadic peripheries provides a productive terrain on which to think about social inequality and the meaning of reproductive justice. The book contributes to a growing area of research on the global politics of reproduction and marks one of the first anthropological demographic studies of Bedouin in the Middle East. Fundamental questions addressed in this study, which pave the way toward broader understanding of socioeconomic disparities in reproduction and survivorship, include: Have the Bedouin and other nomadic groups experienced hierarchical class formation and class distinctions in demographic behavior similar to those found in rural/semirural peasant communities of Europe and Asia? How do local structures of class, kinship, and gender articulate with Bedouin fertility and health? How pervasive is the demographic gap between better-off and worse-off groups within localities and nations? How have some societies managed to escape the three-pronged Malthusian trap of poverty, high fertility, and high mortality? In what ways should conventional views of reproductive justice and liberty be modified to include Bedouin women and other women of color on the interstices of state societies?

Outline of Book Chapters

Fertile Bonds takes up questions of class, kinship, and gender in Bedouin communities with the aim of understanding how reproductive and health inequalities are structured locally and across transnational boundaries. My theoretical approach is best described as political economy of biodemography infused with critical notions of spatiotemporality, structure-agency, and social justice. The critical approach that is advanced challenges the anchoring of reproduction in biology and offers alternative ways of conceptualizing the relationship between nature and nurture.

Chapters 2–6 locate Bedouin women's reproductive lives within a political economy of class, kinship, and gender framework that counters a number of commonplace demographic misconceptions of Arab societies as beset by persistently high fertility, high levels of polygyny, and close-kin marriage practices that are oppressive of women. The chapters identify historically changing regimes of production and reproduction in Bedouin society—changes which have given rise to unique work- and demographic-related experiences among different Bedouin age or birth cohorts. Much of the discussion in these chapters is centered on older Bedouin generations who have lived through the economic transition from nomadic pastoralism to a more peasantized and proletarianized social economy. However, when comparing the life experiences of married Bedouin women 40 years of age and older to their younger married counterparts under 40 years of age (based on their ages in 2000), a related set of differences are discernable in their techno-economic relations, mobility and settlement patterns, age-specific fertility rates, family size preferences, and notions of companionate love within marriage. These intercohort differences are the result of a historical process of de-pastoralization (a process as of yet incomplete) and the concomitant push toward peasant farming and wage labor. I begin in chapter 2 by providing a historical overview of the transition from nomadic pastoralism to a more sedentary agrarian lifestyle among the Bedouin—a transition that has occurred over the course of the twentieth and twenty-first centuries, but with increasing rapidity over the last five decades. Microhistorical estimates are used to situate high and falling Bedouin fertility in local context and in relation to the broader political-economic context of demographic transition in the Arab world.

In chapter 3, I examine the cultural and demographic articulation of social-status hierarchies of class and occupation. Most of the empirical support for social-status differences in health outcomes is based on macro

North-South and between-country disparities. Less is actually known about demographic disparities between local class or status groups within most countries (particularly those outside of Europe) or how those social disparities in birth and death may have changed over time. Chapter 3 and subsequent chapters attempt to fill a gap in our limited demographic understanding of social inequality in nomadic societies. My assessment of fertility and health in the Bekaa affirms the presence of demographic class distinctions between Bedouin and peasant groups in the region, but refutes the presence of a similar sociodemographic gradient within Bedouin communities. The biodemographic determinants of early mortality in Bedouin communities are also highlighted. Chapter 4 turns to the question of gender inequality. The chapter identifies Western feminist misrepresentations of gender and Third World women's reproduction. High fertility in particular is seen as paradigmatic of women's larger oppression within the family. Estimates of gender-specific early morality are used alongside attitudinal measures of the preferred gender configuration of the family to address issues of gender discrimination and child gender preferences in the Bedouin context. Local narratives are used to provide alternative understandings of the cultural valuation of children and large families, while demographic measures help establish the parameters of variation in Bedouin women's fertility.

Chapter 5 provides a thicker ethnographic interpretation of kinship and the marriage between kin. Making sense of consanguineous marriage requires careful understanding of the process of kinship-making and its articulation with occupation and gender. A structure-agency perspective is applied to kin marriages—one that conveys how social positionality and context inform the marriage actions of individuals. I show how Bedouin, by marrying kin, reproduce the kinship system. Kinship is articulated in and through consanguineous marriage. Bedouin couples employed in wage labor are less likely to enter into first-cousin unions than couples working in either pastoralism or sharecropping occupations. Nevertheless, most married couples from across the occupational spectrum share a broader kinship connection as members of the same tribe. Changing notions of love and intimacy observed among newly married adults are used to infer future trends.

Chapter 6 theoretically situates the study of high Bedouin fertility in the broader Malthusian-Marxist debate on population and poverty. The Bekaa Bedouin are best described as a frontier population on the rural peripheries of capitalist expansion. However, contrary to the expectations of Malthusian theory, high Bedouin fertility is not concomitant with disease, death, and abject poverty. Like Anabaptist Hutterites living in the United States, high fertility in Bedouin communities is found in conjunction with low to moderate mortality, adequate nutrition, and good health. I argue that the Bedouin have escaped the Malthusian dilemma through low levels of consumption, hard labor in a mixed economy that affords access to the means of production, egalitarian practices like food sharing, and partial access to high-quality health care. The future population health challenge for the Bedouin lies not in averting the Malthusian trap but in averting dispossession under consumer capitalism.

Chapters 7 and 8 compare and critically evaluate rural studies on social-class disparities in fertility and health. By drawing on a rich array of ethnographic and microdemographic cases from peasant and nomadic communities around the world, these chapters demonstrate the geohistorical complexities of demographic variation and change. Chapter 7 delves into what is arguably one of the most important contributions to the anthropological and sociological study of demography in the last twenty-five years: the identification of local class/caste and occupational differences in microreproductive behavior in rural Europe and Asia at different stages of demographic transitions. The discussion explicitly engages with diversity across localities in Europe, pointing to how cultural practices, in certain time-space contexts, level out class divisions. Understanding the mechanisms and pathways by which social disparities do or do not translate into demographic differentials is critical to addressing structures of inequality and identifying alternative health systems.

Chapter 8 moves out of peasant communities and back onto the nomadic margins to address a fundamental question that remains unclear: do similar forms of class differentiation shape the demographic experiences of nomadic peoples marginalized from the dominant political-economic structures of the nation-state? By focusing on the demographic experiences of marginal nomadic peoples in the Arab world and other regions, the chapter provides a broader analytical lens from which to examine questions about inequality. While hierarchical social relations and classlike demographic differentials have been found in some pastoral groups, broader comparisons reveal a high degree of reproductive and health equality in nomadic foraging and pastoral communities. These findings challenge the premise that egalitarianism is a myth and open up questions about the romanticization of "primitives." The Euramerican romanticization of Bedouin and other "primitives" as "noble savages" uncorrupted by the temptations of civilization rests on colonial oppositions between civilization/barbarism and modernity/tradition. In addition to European and Euramerican interest in appropriating indigenous practices, the Western penchant for "primitives" is bound up with the contestation of values in the dominant culture. Idealized sentiments toward the "primitive" are more common in "low" culture. Anthropologists are often hesitant to express views that appear to be too favorable, lest they be perceived as nonobjective or, worse, as naïve, fawning, utopian, kitschy, new-age romantics. Instead, most opt for either extreme postmodern cynicism (e.g., saying "inequality is universal") or the safe middle ground (e.g., saying "there is a little of this and a little of that").

The final chapter takes stock of what an anthropological demographic study of Bedouin reproduction in Lebanon and the Syria Desert has to say about class, gender, and the demographic divide. Bedouin communities in the Middle East are an appropriate site for probing concepts of equality and women's reproductive liberty, asking not only what these concepts mean, but who they benefit and who they leave out. Stories of birth and death are also stories of class, race, kinship, and gender relations. However, the Bedouin case illustrates that demographic realities are uneven in time and place; hence, the need to geographically and historically situate accounts of reproductive difference.

The foregoing chapters taken together also raise questions about how to integrate biopolitics and culture into discussions of stratified reproduction. Critical researchers often find that biological differences originate in the social order and are a product of social structure. Social forces under the guise of biology work to create and perpetuate classism and racism. Although Malthus recognized the existence of class realities, he ultimately naturalized poverty, in effect, denying the social underpinnings of demographic behavior. Malthusian theory has exerted considerable influence on Darwinism, Social Darwinism, and eugenics. The idea of a Hobbesian struggle for existence in which rampant sexual procreation would outstrip the production of food, exposing certain elements of society (i.e., the poor "surplus population") to starvation and Malthusian catastrophe left the door open for scientific classism and racism. More than 200 years after the publication of Malthus's *An Essay on the Principle of Population*, it remains a fundamental challenge for social and natural scientists to understand human demographic events without glossing over or naturalizing the social determinants of inequality. Similarly, a pervasive feature of public discourses in the imperial metropole is the use of "culture" to explain reproductive and health differences. Critical medical anthropologists have problematized such accounts for "conflating structural violence and cultural difference," to use anthropologist and physician Paul Farmer's phrase. Thus, far from being distinct, the biologizing and culturalizing of poverty and human suffering demonstrate that nature-nurture arguments are often correlatives—opposite sides of the same coin. A critical analysis of the social facts of birth and death requires re-imagining the dialectic between nature and nurture, biology and culture, and their articulation with power. Culture is malleable, not monolithic, which implies that cultural forms can be used to both legitimate and destabilize power. With the foregoing discussion in mind, I turn to spell out in more detail the theoretical currents that have shaped the book.

Critical Theory and Social Justice

Demographic understanding, like all forms of social-scientific understanding, proceeds with the asking of questions. In his classic work *Historians' Fallacies*, David Hackett Fischer observes that social inquiry generally follows one of the following three patterns: it occasionally consists of attempts to learn "everything about everything"; it sometimes consists of attempts to learn "something about everything"; and it most often consists of attempts to learn "everything about something." Fischer rejects all three as impossible quests and suggests that the only realistic aim is to learn "something about something."[12] Works that straddle disciplines—in this case, anthropology and demography as well as cultural and biological anthropology—are particularly vulnerable to Fischer's third charge of trying to learn "everything about something" or, worse, "everything about everything." Even if we adopt a narrower focus on the analysis and interpretation of demographic disparities in reproductive and health outcomes, we are still left with the question of how to interpret those demographic facts. Are demographic events best seen as outcomes of social or biological processes?

The modern debate over the role of biological versus social forces in explaining demographic differentiation can be traced to Malthus's famous essay, first published in 1798. The principle of population advanced by Malthus is that all life tends to grow "beyond the nourishment prepared for it" and therefore a "strong check on population from the difficulty of acquiring food, must constantly be in operation."[13] Malthus saw high fertility—induced by a biological sexual urge in human beings—as a destructive force that threatens economic well-being, health, and survival. However, more than just a negative force, Malthus regarded poverty as the natural plight of the poor, who, because of their "innate" moral passions, were believed to be incapable of exercising restraint from early marriage and sexual gratification before marriage.[14] Karl Marx and Friedrich Engels, well-known critics of Malthus on the other side of the debate, emphasized the role of exploitative and poorly organized economies in fueling poverty, misery, and population growth. Instead of attributing the plight of the poor to the "natural law" of population, Marx recognized socially and historically specific "laws" of population. Marx and Engels laid the initial foundations for rejecting simplistic economic or bioecological scarcity arguments and paved the way toward more spatially and historically contingent political-economic analysis. However, Marxist approaches in the social sciences do not provide specific guidelines on how to integrate bioecological forces into the study of population. Malthusianism/neo-Malthusianism, on the other hand, places strong emphasis on the bioecological causes and consequences of population growth, but often does so in ways that naturalize nurture and demonstrate little compassion for the social struggles of peoples in colonial and imperial situations both historically and at present.

More recently, anthropologists have proclaimed the need for a less conflicted articulation between biology, history, and politics. As Paul Farmer states, "Complex biosocial phenomena are the focus of most anthropological inquiries, and yet the integration of history, political economy, and biology remains lacking in contemporary anthropology or sociology."[15] Similarly, upon reviewing 3,264 articles that appeared in the *American Anthropologist (AA)* from 1899–1998 and designating those he deemed to be "holistic," Robert Borofsky found that only 9.5 percent of all articles published in the *AA* over a hundred-year period possess substantive subfield collaboration, despite a century of anthropologists extolling the virtues of holistic approaches.[16] The volume *Building a New Biocultural Synthesis*, by Alan Goodman and Thomas Leatherman, was a pioneering attempt to address the lack of such intradisciplinary collaboration in anthropology.[17] These new efforts to integrate biological with political-economic perspectives as part of the new biocultural synthesis have begun to reveal how social inequalities shape human biology in prehistoric, historical, and contemporary populations.

While attempts to bring critical theory to the field of biology are relatively recent, the initial effort to develop a critical interpretation of health within (sociocultural) medical anthropology began in the 1970s. In 1982, the field was officially designated critical medical anthropology (CMA) and became virtually synonymous with a political-economy-of-health perspective.[18] The field of anthropological demography, formally designated fifteen years later, in 1997, shares considerable theoretical content with CMA. Critical perspectives in both fields—medical anthropology and anthropological demography—seek to understand demographic and health issues within the context of broader institutional forces—those operating at national and global levels of human social organization and over broad stretches of time.

Identifying strands of allegiance within and between fields is somewhat impressionistic and certainly open to contestation, but I would also point to a differentially shared recognition within CMA and anthropological demography that an *empirically* informed critical theory is a worthwhile social-scientific endeavor.[19] Empirical studies can benefit from the counsel of critical theory. The reverse is also true, as critical theory can be refined and reformulated as empirical research warrants. There is no shortage of critical studies in either CMA or anthropological demography. However, sociocultural anthropological attempts to forge a critical *biocultural* alliance are less apparent, especially in anthropological demography. In its short history as a discipline, anthropological demography has regularly incorporated a public-health focus, but has struggled to incorporate contributions from biodemography.[20] Cross-disciplinary efforts to build a new biocultural synthesis have been met with skepticism from critics on both sides, but sociocultural anthropologists are generally more apprehensive. Much of the skepticism between biological and sociocultural subfields of anthropology stems from long-standing epistemological and methodological differences, which are laced with political and emotional content. One need only recall the distorted Darwinism used to legitimize racist and eugenicist social policies to appreciate the seriousness of such concerns. The dangers of misapplying biology to the study of human behavior should serve as a caveat to research, as biological anthropologist Melvin Konner warns in *The Tangled Wing*: "it would be far better for behavioral biology to disappear from view than to be applied as carelessly, as stupidly and as destructively as it has been in the past."[21] A critical approach is best equipped to engage in biocultural analysis that is sensitive to the dangers of domination and oppression in human societies. By shedding light on the normalization and naturalization of power within both cultural and biological subfields, a critical approach allows for a different reading of demographic facts. Social relations of class, race, and gender are often intimately linked to the biopolitical exercise of power.

Integrating principles from biology (physiology and evolutionary processes such as natural selection) and culture (structures of meaning and their articulation with structures of power and legitimation) does not simply mean "mix and stir." Instead, as social scientists, we have to do a better job of specifying the scale in time and space to which a given theory refers, which also means understanding the limitations of each theory. No one theory can do it all. Critical inquiry is pluralistic and interdisciplinary in its outlook without being chaotic or indiscriminate. By taking pluralism and complexity into account, critical theory moves away from seeking a single unifying theory[22] and toward employing different theories in a manner mindful of history and geography. Critical or political-economic approaches in demography are based on the recognition that understanding microreproductive behavior requires simultaneous attention to proximate mechanisms (including biological mechanisms) and more remote structures and processes—both structure and agency.[23] Only broader-level analysis (usually involving larger areas or longer periods of time) can reveal why a demographic pattern exists in the first place.

Another advantage of critical theory is that it provides some guidance for human action—a basis from which to contemplate the righting of wrongs. Critical theory is self-reflective and intersubjectively engaged, embracing the broader goal of freedom from domination. As David Macey states, "The object of a critical theory such as Marxism is to supply the knowledge of the necessity of transforming the present social order into a classless society. It does not, however, predict the inevitability of that transformation and merely points to what *ought* to be done rather than to what *will* happen."[24] Critical theory provides emancipatory knowledge, thereby giving social actors the tools they need to confront classism, racism, sexism, social Darwinism, and eugenicism.

Because the theories used to combat oppression in human societies may themselves serve as instruments of domination and control (in spite of the intentions of their creators), critical theory demands a critical appraisal of critical theory itself. Gayatri Spivak has observed that inherent in the contemporary notion of "human rights" and "the white man's burden" is the imprint of social Darwinism: "the fittest must shoulder the burden of righting the wrongs of the unfit."[25] Although Western countries serve as the ideological impetus behind "human rights" and "development" as well as the source of funding, training, and pressure, a local colonial class of capitalists and intellectuals was created in the postcolonial countries of the Third World, some of the descendants of whom became the educated middle-class advocates of "human rights" today.

Reproductive-rights advocates have espoused an agenda that looks an awful lot like the old social Darwinism and Galtonian eugenicism—the ideological bulwarks of the population-control movement. Population aid has always been oriented toward population control as opposed to women's health and economic initiatives.[26] Overpopulation rhetoric and policy have traditionally focused on avoiding the "dangers" of polluting the planet with too many people, particularly the wrong kind of people. In spite of the global decline in fertility, the need to control population is seen as especially urgent in the context of plunging birth rates in Europe and its overseas offshoots (e.g., Canada and Australia). The difference today is that the population problem is increasingly articulated in terms of an implosion in the global North as opposed to an explosion in the global South. Positive eugenics (promoting the population of the "racially fit") has superseded negative eugenics (curbing the population of the "racially unfit").

In his groundbreaking global history of the population-control movement, Matthew Connelly heralds 1994 as the year, and the UN-sponsored International Conference on Population and Development (ICPD) held in Cairo as the event, that marked the defeat of population control as a global movement and the triumph of a reproductive-rights and health agenda. Gone were mandates for reducing population growth. In their place were calls pioneered by the international women's movement to improve the lot of women. A new global consensus emerged that women have the right to exercise control over their own bodies and reproductive lives without coercion or manipulation. Progressive notions of gender equality, equity, and empowerment were introduced. The political focus shifted away from target levels of population toward an individual-level model with women's rights, health, and status at the center. At the same time that Connelly celebrates the triumph of reproductive rights, he warns of the emergence of unforeseen forms of power in the future, particularly as privileged classes increasingly seek genetic counseling, IVF, international adoption, surrogacy, and "egg donation"—what Connelly refers to as the "privatization of population control."[27] However, we are not simply dealing with new and unforeseen dangers that might arise in the near future, but ongoing struggles that exist here and now. The central problem is itself a mainstay of Western feminism: neoliberal capitalism.

Here again, characterizations of low fertility set against the backdrop of high fertility are revealing. Connelly observes that lower fertility rates worldwide correspond with higher rates of literacy and education among women. In explaining this pattern, Connelly further asserts that these women "have had an education and thus more opportunities to accomplish things besides bearing children."[28] The problematic assumption here is that poor rural women with no formal schooling and no mastery of written forms of communication have accomplished little in their lives other than bearing and raising children (which is no minor accomplishment). Aside from the social failure to acknowledge the economic contribution of women's unpaid domestic labor, there is the related failure to recognize that many poor rural women with children also engage in paid work and play multiple social roles in their communities. What we have is the implicit stereotype of a rural, illiterate, poor, barefoot and pregnant woman who needs to be "rescued." But even here neoliberalism cannot help her, as the capitalist desire to get ahead entails instrumental treatment of other persons. Connelly acknowledges: "Many [middle/upper middle class] parents already realize, for instance, that their choices between work and family, however difficult, would be impossible without the aid of poor women who have no choice but to leave their own families behind."[29] And herein lies the problem: the collusion between capitalist modernization, feminism, and racism. (After all, these poor women are mostly women of color.) Prosperity of the few is ineluctably linked to the exploitation of the many.

We know that many wrongs have been committed in the name of justice, freedom, and human rights. Just as colonialism and imperialism enjoin the "civilized" world to "liberate" Arab-Muslim women, the population-control and reproductive-rights movements have their own colonial mandate to "rescue" poor rural women in the global South from high fertility. The liberation-cum-control of women's reproduction remains central to the civilizing mission of modernity. High and "uncontrolled" fertility continue to be depicted as a "problem" to be solved. But this does not mean that we should abandon the cause for justice. Rather, concepts of reproductive justice and liberty need to be revised to accommodate the reproductive experiences of women in marginalized Third World and Fourth World[30] communities. A central pillar of reproductive justice involves bridging class, race, and gender divides, but must do so in ways that are not oppressive to poor peoples in the global South and metropole. The condemnation of high birth rates disparages the reproduction of poor rural women of color and perpetuates what bell hooks denotes "white capitalist patriarchy."[31]

Class, race, and gender are indispensible tools for social analysis and social change—linked to one another and to the concept of culture. Culture has taken on global significance as nineteenth-century notions of race and race wars have given way to culture and clash of cultures. Racism is increasingly articulated in terms of culture. Culture is the new kid on the block to be sketched and measured—the phrenology used to decipher the "other." Take for example a *New York Times* article entitled "A Hunt for Genes that Betrayed a Desert People," which describes Bedouin intermarriage as a social and biological tragedy born out of despotic tradition: "Until recently their ancestors were nomads who roamed the deserts of the Middle East and, as tradition dictated, often married cousins. Marrying within the family helped strengthen bonds among extended families struggling to survive the desert. But after centuries this custom of intermarriage has had devastating genetic effects."[32] The article goes on to describe the social suffering of the family due to cultural tradition, but ultimately finds "hope" in genetic testing and counseling. The reader is assured that the Bedouin will lead "better lives" as a result of modern genetic research. (There is no mention of the devastating impacts of colonial violence in the Negev.) In the context of genetically defective Bedouin lives, "better" means less. We are told that "under Islam a woman can abort a fetus up to four months for health reasons."[33] The message of the article is clear: have fewer babies, particularly genetically defective Bedouin babies—a directive that happens to coincide with the interests of the occupying Zionist entity.

What is remarkable is the extent to which culture fills in for race,[34] inscribing differences into human bodies that are difficult to dislodge and give rise to pathologies. Archaic culture leaves a lasting biological mark. The "hunt for genes" turns up a culture that is not so well-designed and better weeded-out. Bedouin culture—depicted as "static" and "atavistic"—is believed to be at the crux of societal and health problems. Culture is frequently deemed to be at the root of one "crisis" or another. Arabs and Arab civilization have long been characterized as "backward," "decadent," and crisis-prone. Oriental culture, language, and traditions—in effect, the sum total of cultural life, including Islam itself—were believed to be in crisis/decline/fall as a result of centuries of Ottoman rule. There is considerable overlap in the set of ideas contained within the population paradigm and Orientalism. The latter can be understood as a form of white supremacy in which European colonial powers developed a self-justifying academic field of study and mode of discourse on the Orient (supported by colonial institutions, bureaucracies, and military force) that portrayed peoples and societies of those lands as "exotic," dangerous, "homogenous," "unchanging," and, above all, "inferior."[35] Because the Orient was seen as incapable not only of representing itself but also of modernizing, liberating, or "civilizing" itself, the "civilizing" process had to be overseen by European and, later, American colonizers.

Orientalist caricatures, depicting Arabs as camel-riding, violent, and "uncivilized," take on a different racial intonation when applied to Bedouin tribal peoples. Tribal Fourth World peoples have all too frequently been relegated to a "lower" stage of humanity's evolutionary development. Anthropology has long wrestled with these issues of primitivism and cultural racism, given its focus on tribal and ethnic peoples, civilized states, and the relationship between them. Evidence of cultural imperialism at work is perhaps nowhere more apparent than in writings on tribal peoples frequently depicted as ignoble/noble savages. But these are some of the challenges of doing anthropology in tribal nomadic and ex-nomadic communities. Edward Said once remarked on the important legacy of his work for the discipline of anthropology: "In anthropology in particular, it raised the question of what it means when an entire science is based upon unequal power between two cultures."[36] Said explicitly acknowledged that his work does not provide an understanding of what Middle Eastern peoples are actually like; he left the task of representing the actualities and varieties of cultural life in the Middle East to other scholars. Before proceeding to the cultural and demographic realities of Bedouin life in the chapters that follow, I pause to consider the methodology used to carry out the present study.

Doing Critical Demographic and Ethnographic Research

Research is an iterative back-and-forth process. Experience often warrants revision, refinement, and even rejection of theories and methods. When I arrived in the Bekaa in 2000, my research was strongly informed by (uncritical) Marxist/neo-Marxist views on rich-poor class divisions articulated in and through demographic conjunctures. After only two months in the Bekaa, I remember calling my husband at the time to tell him that class, gender, and social positionality were far more complex than my initial presuppositions allowed. I knew that I was off about so much. Listening to taped interviews in the field often made me cringe, as it was obvious from my importunate questioning that I was probing for responses that conformed to my own hegemonic views on class and gender, not to mention my dismissal of kinship. It was only after a few months that I began to listen and make reasonable connections and inferences coherent with my experiences in the field. It took me many years of reflection, writing, and hesitation before I was comfortable collecting my thoughts together in a book. Some insights came during fieldwork and others came years later. We know that anthropological representations of Arab women, marriage, family life, etc. can be lifted from their proper ethnographic context and used to support colonial and imperial agendas. As anthropologists, we often unwittingly reproduce versions of colonial assumptions in our ethnographic writing. In our efforts to come to terms with the destructive legacies of colonialism and imperialism, there is a corollary danger that anthropologists of the Middle East may take the opposite tack of valorizing Arab peoples. Opposites come together at this juncture, leading to caricaturelike representations of bad Arab versus good Arab.

Mounting an effective challenge against essentializing trends in anthropology means sharpening our critical thinking and writing. Whenever possible, we must try to spatially and historically contextualize relations of power and meaning (including the power relation between those who represent and those who are represented); confront the constructivist tensions between biology, culture, and power; identify conceptual-empirical contributions, as well as gaps in our knowledge; and winnow out oversimplifications and assertions that lack proof. In the chapters that follow, I draw from critical theory to forge an empirically sound demographic study of Bedouin in rural Lebanon. The anthropological study of demography in marginalized nomadic communities has the potential to rewrite our understandings of class, kinship, gender, and social justice.

To capture the multiple contexts of Bedouin reproduction and health experiences, I use a combination of ethnographic, biodemographic, and microhistorical methods. Reproductive-history and work-history interviews form the primary basis of the book's demographic and economic findings. The reproductive- and work-history interviews are highly detailed, consisting of semi-structured questions on production and reproduction in Bedouin society. All interviews were conducted in Arabic without the assistance of a translator. The need to establish rapport and allow sufficient time for introductions and expressions of hospitality meant that semi-structured reproductive- and work-history interviews were often conducted half an hour or more after arriving at each home. Many of the homes visited were shacks and tents in small, more temporary settlements and enclaves. Reproductive- and work-history interviews themselves took, on average, slightly over an hour to complete. Bedouin women and men appeared to enjoy discussing their reproductive and productive lives. I was fortunate not to be turned away by anyone, although I did reschedule several interviews. Occasional return visits for cross-checking and follow-up of participant responses were also required. Age estimation and dating of births/deaths proved to be more difficult among older women. I devoted considerable time to developing a local event calendar to help reduce age-estimation errors.[37] The calendar was based on political events (e.g., uprisings, deaths of political leaders, transfers of political power), well-known battles during the Lebanese Civil War (1975–91), Zionist military attacks and occupations, and even snowstorms.[38]

Direct reproductive histories were collected in 2000–2001 from a systematic random sample of 240 ever-married Bedouin women between the ages of fifteen and fifty-four residing in the Bekaa Valley. Reproductive histories were also completed with 108 of the women's spouses. (The living husbands of Bedouin women were interviewed if they were present at the time of my visit[s] to their household.) Reproductive histories were used to derive estimates of fertility, perinatal mortality (stillbirths and miscarriages), and postnatal infant and child mortality.[39] In addition, reproductive histories provide information on marital histories of individuals (separation, divorce, or widowhood) and local marriage systems (patriparallel cousin marriage, exchange marriage, and polygyny). To obtain further information on Bedouin nutritional and health status, anthropometric measurements of height (cm) and weight (kg) were taken from 240 Bedouin women (and seventeen Bedouin men) in 2000–2001. Measures of skinfold thicknesses (mm) at the triceps and subscapula as well as mid-upper arm circumferences (cm) were only taken from Bedouin women in 2000–2001.[40]

In 2007, I decided to enlarge my sample of postreproductive women to get a better picture of high fertility among the older generation of Bedouin women. The forty-one additional reproductive histories with postmeno-pausal women (who had completed their childbearing) were not based on a randomly selected sample. Instead, I used a variation of the family-reg-istration method. I visited more than six Bedouin enclaves from different regions in the Bekaa. From those, I selected one or two neighborhoods or streets and interviewed all of the postreproductive women from those ar-eas. The forty-one Bedouin women interviewed in 2007 belong to the same birth cohorts as postreproductive women interviewed in 2000 (1946–1960), with the exception of five women who belong to a birth cohort four years older (born between 1942 and 1945). In total, I completed 281 reproductive-history interviews with Bedouin women. To derive historical estimates of Bedouin fertility, I conducted indirect reproductive-history interviews with a subsample of 160 women (out of 240 women interviewed in 2000) whose mothers were postreproductive either at the time of their death or at the time of the interview (see chapter 2 for a discussion of the method employed and the results).

In conjunction with direct reproductive-history interviews, direct work-history interviews were completed with 281 women and 108 of their spouses. I used work histories to determine socioeconomic designations. Some of the socioeconomic measures derived include primary occupation or domi-nant local mode of production since a couple's marriage, marital (or other) inheritance, and wealth index of the basic means of production.[41] Indirect work histories—that is, individuals who reported on their parents' occu-pational history—were obtained in 2000–2001 from 240 Bedouin women (224 of which were complete) in order to better characterize changes in the Bedouin economic structure through time. Ethnographic methods—par-ticipant observation and oral histories with a subsample of 15 women and 10 men—were used to explore the meaning of marriage and economic and family life among the Bedouin. Because oral histories were highly open-ended and flexible, each oral-history interview had a slightly different word-ing of questions, emphasis, direction, and tempo. In the summer of 2007, I conducted an additional five semi-structured interviews with newly mar-ried couples. My research assistant transcribed most of the taped interviews into Arabic; however all of the Arabic-to-English transcriptions and Arabic-to-English translations are my own. Personal, family, and tribal names were generally omitted or changed to protect participant privacy and maintain confidentiality. However, some personal names were left as is to accommodate participants who did not wish to have their identities disguised or concealed.

Government and nongovernment sources (e.g., creditors' books, maternal- and child-health surveys from Lebanon and neighboring Middle Eastern countries, and Lebanese Ministry of Agriculture statistics) were used to complement reproductive histories and work histories as well as further understand Bedouin economic ties to peasant society. Overall, the book is based on almost two years of ethnographic and demographic fieldwork in rural Bedouin communities of the Bekaa Valley, Lebanon and the Syrian Desert—four months of preliminary research in 1998, fifteen months between 2000 and 2001, and three months during the summer of 2007.

Establishing Relationships

As a native Lebanese anthropologist, I enjoyed several advantages in terms of language familiarity and religious commonality with my Bedouin interlocutors. However, it should be added that native identity confers no absolute or fixed "insider" advantages in doing research. Self-perception and others' perceptions of us can shift with context and community setting.[42] Bedouin peasant-class tensions and divisions influenced my own decision, as a native non-Bedouin Arab, not to enlist the assistance of peasant farmers in establishing contacts within Bedouin village communities. Peasant-class devaluation of Bedouin is ubiquitous. Since I did not share the same sentiments, and did not want to be perceived as such, I ended up establishing contacts on my own in each Bedouin village or neighborhood.

At the beginning of my fieldwork, I was uncertain as to how well this would work. My male research assistant, who is of mixed Bedouin and peasant ancestry, accompanied me on some of these initial research visits, although I did most of the talking. A crucial part of building trust involved not only explaining my academic research as a doctoral student but also my personal biography as a second-generation member of the Lebanese diaspora with family ties to my home country. My married life and my relationship with my in-laws was a topic of some interest to my Bedouin interlocutors, as was my then husband's absence in the field. (My husband at the time was abroad completing graduate study in the United States.) A few Bedouin men, and more than a few peasant men from the village of my former spouse, teased that my husband had probably paired up with a second wife in America, while others reproached him in absentia for not being there to protect his wife. I do not recall anyone pointedly asking me about my religious faith in 2000–2001. Only one pious middle-aged Bedouin man asked me why I was not veiled, citing the book and sunna as to the dangers of women's uncovering, particularly uncovered hair. I responded by assuring him that those women most definitely had better hair and that there was little danger of mine inducing a call to arms. He laughed easily, which is not surprising, seeing that Bekaa Bedouin have a warm sense of humor.

I would describe my conversations with Bekaa Bedouin women and men as candid, open, and relaxed. We discussed childbearing, marriage, divorce, honor, modesty, and politics. I felt little need to engage in dissimulation commonly reported in fieldwork. Much has been made of tensions centered around the topic of sexuality in the writings of women anthropologists in the Middle East. Being married made it easier to ask questions of other married women about sexual intimacy, but sometimes my own modesty (and youth in 2000–2001) made it difficult for me not to feel like I was prying. Most incongruities stemmed from interchanges over political leanings. About 10 percent of Bedouins, somewhere around ten thousand to twelve thousand, were granted citizenship under Rafiq Hariri, the assassinated former prime minister. The few who were granted citizenship were adult men and women. In other words, "citizenship" was granted to individual males and females. The fact that many Bedouin adults were married and had children was discounted. The outcome has been that most Bedouin citizens are stateless and have only partial access to national primary health-care facilities[43] (see chapter 3). Nevertheless, owing to this minimal conferral of "citizenship" and to their identity as Sunni Muslims, several of my Bedouin interlocutors expressed sympathies with the Sunni-led March 14th coalition over the opposition led by Hizbullah and the former General Michel Aoun, Christian leader of the Free Patriotic Movement—a movement that enjoyed the support of the majority of the Christian population in Lebanon at the time of my research. I felt very comfortable sharing my own outspoken views on politics, marriage, and family life, as I felt genuine affection for and developed close ties to Bedouin families in Lebanon and Syria.

Having family connections in the Bekaa Valley (my now ex-husband's family resides there) made the logistics of research easier. There were also some disadvantages, as obligations to family sometimes intruded on research. Personal tensions also surfaced over the derogation of Bedouin by peasant visitors and neighbors. My former affines were aware of my research plans, seeing that I had decided to work with Bedouin in the Bekaa long before I was married. Our paths (the Bekaa Bedouin and I) first crossed in the winter of 1994 as I saw families assembled together in their black goat-haired tents in the village of Mansoura. In 1998, I spent four months in the Bekaa conducting preliminary ethnographic research for my dissertation in anthropology at the University of Georgia. Upon receiving grant funding, I returned in 2000–2001 for fifteen months to complete my dissertation research. I was married during the entire duration of my fieldwork in 2000–2001. My Arab in-laws' residence served as my primary home base. In time, as I became better acquainted personally with Bedouin women and their families, I divided my time between three host families from different villages and tribes in the region. When I returned to the Bekaa for a three-month follow-up research trip in the summer of 2007, I was divorced and so divided my stay between my ex-husband's sister's family and a Bedouin family with whom I had established a close friendship.

I observed many changes on my return trip to the Bekaa in 2007, one of the most noticeable of which was war-induced suffering. It is difficult to describe what it is like doing research in the aftermath of war. The economic suffering endured by Bedouin families (and other families in the region) during and after the Israeli war on Lebanon in July 2006 is somewhat easier to measure than the emotional pain. Several families whom I visited in 2007 had friends and relatives who lost their lives during the war. However, by far the most common losses reported were livestock and crop-related damages. Many Bedouin families saw their livestock perish, either due to fire from direct bombings or to an inability to access feed. Crop losses were also sustained from having to leave crops unattended during the military bombardments. One of the most important long-term effects of the 2006 war appears to be unemployment. Loss of labor opportunities can be attributed to direct and indirect shocks from damage to land, livestock, and public infrastructure (electrical facilities, irrigation infrastructure, Qaraoun Dam and packing stations as well as cold-storage facilities in the Bekaa).[44] Many Bedouin agropastoral families in 2007 were struggling to recover from losses and debt incurred from the devastation. These struggles are only the most recent in what has been a long and painful history of economic recovery from decades of civil war, Syrian occupation, and ongoing United States–backed Zionist colonial wars/invasions. In the ten-plus years that I have spent visiting the Bekaa for research and personal reasons, I have never been asked by so many people as often as I was in 2007 if I could help them migrate and locate work outside of Lebanon. The long-term economic and population health impacts of the recent war (including the impacts of bomb-induced water, soil, and crop contamination) await future study.

The most visible changes I observed in 2007 were those related to the physical structure and population size of Bedouin villages. Bedouin villages and neighborhoods in the Bekaa are relatively young (see chapter 2). The unfinished and sparsely furnished quality of Bedouin homes stands out in contrast to those found in peasant villages and towns. Poorer Bedouin families, who can ill afford to purchase land and build permanent homes, reside in temporary tin shacks. At the time of my fieldwork in 2000, 4.5 percent of Bedouins lived in tents, 6.7 percent in shacks, 8.8 percent in combined tent and house dwellings, and 80 percent lived in stone/cement houses. When I returned about six years later in 2007, I noticed that several joint families consisting of married brothers and their children had splintered off into separate households. The costs of sedentary life—including home construction, food costs, utilities, transportation, and schooling—could be seen and felt everywhere. And yet, compared with 2000, the homes of middle-class Bedouin families had more modern touches. Many were laid with marble-tiled flooring and equipped with store-bought furniture. Access to some Bedouin villages also improved. A few of the already existing roads had been paved, and these same villages had completed construction on mosques and schools. Bedouin villages had obviously grown in size. Given a doubling time of approximately twelve years, villages were almost 50 percent larger than I found them in 2000–2001. The next chapter takes a closer look at the major economic and demographic transformations that took place in Bedouin society over the course of the twentieth and early twenty-first centuries.

2

Nomadic Lives in Transition

Bedouin tribal nomadism has been altered by processes similar to those affecting pastoralists everywhere. Bedouin nomadic movements in search of pasture and water for their sheep and goats have been impacted by the solidification of national boundaries, changes in systems of land tenure, commoditization of the livestock economy, the expansion of industrial agriculture, the mechanization of transport, urbanization, and population growth. Most Bedouins residing in the Bekaa Valley, Lebanon, today live in permanent or semipermanent structures and rely on farming for their livelihoods. Only a fraction of the population—roughly one-quarter—continues to rely on pastoralism. In the recent past, the situation was reversed, with most families working as pastoralists. Pastoral households migrated as a unit from winter to spring pastures, as family members herded the sheep and camels transported their tents and possessions.[1] Rḥayla, a Bedouin woman in her mid-fifties in 2000, remembers what life was like when she and her family lived as pastoral nomads:

> Our family had sheep, camels, and horses. We milked the sheep and "shook up" [churned] the milk to make *samn* (clarified butter, or ghee). We made dried yogurt-cheese and boys herded the sheep and returned [to camp]. The men carried coffee and we lived in goat-hair tents, not stone houses. All day long we had visitors, [served] coffee and tea . . . and [felt] *kayf* (pleasure) and *basṭ* (happiness). You should have seen the camels that we dressed and decorated—and the horses were decorated too. My family also raised gazelles. We had ten gazelles at the [tent] house and decorated them all. We used to pour milk for them . . . Our family had over one thousand sheep [shared between three brothers and their families]. My parents had eight boys and me [a girl]. I am the second oldest. . . .
>
> We moved over seven times per year. We moved a lot. If we stayed twenty days or one month in the same area—oh "gentle one" [one of the Lord's many names]—we would go crazy and say "This land is no

good anymore; it's time to move." Baalbek, Jib Janine, and the land on the border with Syria are [the areas] where we grazed our flocks. There was no farmland in the winter, just *barriyya* (open country or wild land) in the Syrian Desert where we grazed the sheep. We migrated to the Syrian border or the Syrian Desert in the winter. At the beginning of the summer at the time of the harvest, we came to Baalbek and then later traveled to the Marj. When the wheat harvest was over [in Baalbek], we sought [residues from] other crops: onions, potatoes, garlic, lima beans, and chickpeas. Sometimes we did not pay money for grazing but exchanged milk [with peasant farmers] instead . . . My father had many friends from Baalbek who would visit for lunch. They ate *lazkiyyī* (pancakes) in the summer; they slaughtered lamb and made meat pies on the *saj* (convex disc-shaped griddle heated from below by wood fire) [served] with laban and garlic. . . .

We [our camping unit] did not split up until there were thirty-five men in the camp. It got too big—boys and girls and [young] children. Each son had his inheritance. My father split from his brothers in 1962. He split from his brothers when he was an old man. We could not make enough bread to keep up [with the needs of the joint family]. My family purchased land in the 1960s. Land was 100 [Lebanese] liras per dunum in the Marj. My family bought land and forgot about it. We did not know where it was . . . When I was fifteen years old, my family stopped going to the Syrian Desert. We went to the Qaa [on the border of Syria] and came back to the Bekaa. There was no suq in the Marj [located in West Bekaa]. I do not remember it [being there]. There was a suq in Ghazieh [in south Lebanon]. A Lebanese merchant would come and we would sell him sheep—thirty at a time. He would buy them for their wool. We received lots of visitors. My family slaughtered sheep for guests about three times per week. We baked bread every day. There were other Bedouin families with their tents, about twenty tents for one Bedouin family and twenty tents [that belonged] to another [camping unit]. We used to invite each other . . .

From the above passage, it is clear that the Bekaa Bedouin have been heavily reliant on agricultural communities and, hence, are best described as agropastoralists. (However, I continue to use the term "pastoralists" to underscore the distinction between them and Bedouins involved primarily in agricultural production.) Close agnatic kin, mostly brothers or patriparallel cousins, shared a camp and collectively herded livestock, which were individually owned. Long-distance horizontal migration in the winter was coupled with short-distance vertical transhumance between high mountain pastures in the spring and lowland agricultural fields during the summer months.

Traditional winter grazing lands were east of Homs (in the direction of Palmyra) in the Syrian Desert. The Syrian Desert extends north from the Nafud Desert in Saudi Arabia and comprises western Iraq, eastern Jordan, and southeastern Syria. The Syrian Desert is covered with grass and scrub vegetation, which are used extensively for pasture by both nomadic and seminomadic herders. The Arabic word *Badu*, or Bedouin, means an inhabitant of "*al-bādiya*," or the semidesert steppe located between the cultivated lands on the eastern Mediterranean coast and the fertile Euphrates River Valley. These traditional winter pastures are in bloom from early January up until March. In oral histories, Bedouin women estimated that their camping units in Syria (which consisted of twenty to thirty household units) moved at least once every two weeks or so. The lambing of the flock occurred in February or March. Bedouin families who did not migrate to these distant winter pastures headed to the northern caves of the Qaa to shelter their sheep from the cold wet winter in the Bekaa. During April to early May, tribes began moving back toward the Bekaa Valley. Bedouins camped in scattered and remote areas along the Anti-Lebanon Mountains where their sheep could graze on natural pastures. Toward the close of the spring season, arrangements were made between household heads and individual farmers in the Bekaa, whereby Bedouin flocks could graze on the stubble of harvested fields and in turn fertilize the farmer's fields with sheep manure. The economic arrangement between Bedouin pastoralists and fellahin in the Bekaa was considered mutually beneficial to both parties. Historically, Bedouins remained in the Bekaa until the winter season (late September to early October), which again marked their movement north or east.[2]

Ethnographic evidence points to close economic ties between Bedouin and peasant groups. In oral histories, Bedouins reported selling milk and milk products to a merchant who periodically visited their camping units to collect milk or *samn* for sweet shops in Beirut. As cheese and dairy factories sprang up in the Bekaa after the 1960s, Bedouins began selling milk to local industries. One Bedouin family, who stopped summering in the Bekaa Valley after 1958 and began to migrate to fertile regions of Syria instead, namely Ghouta and Hauran, similarly reported being visited by a merchant. The rural merchant who came to their tribal camp every year was described as "a pious village man who rides a donkey and carries a stick." He made the yearly rounds, visiting a different tribe each month—roughly four hundred houses per year. The peasant villager was a jack-of-all-trades: a milkman, circumciser, barber, and "dentist" all in one. He rendered a variety of services to his Bedouin clients, including shaving the men, attending to toothaches, and circumcising a group of about thirty boys at a time every two to three years. In exchange for his services, he received milk or *samn* from Bedouin families.

The traditional interdependence between Bedouin and fellah rests on the exchange of food with pastoralists receiving grains and vegetables in return for meat and dairy items. A traditional way of life that involved migration to an arid environment made the preservation of food difficult. Mobility prevents cultivation and storage of large amounts of food among pastoralists, but the summer portion of the migratory cycle brings pastoralists and farmers together. Bedouin pastoralists relied on drying and fermentation to preserve food. Milk and milk products have always been the mainstays of a traditional Bedouin diet. When milk is in season, Bedouin milk twice daily. The morning milk is used to make *samn* and *laban*. Afternoon milk is used to make cheese. Milk and milk products can be preserved for future consumption when milk is not in season. Bedouin ate dried yogurt balls and drank reconstituted dried yogurt by adding water to it. Wheat—in the form of baked bread and *burghul* (cracked wheat)—has always been a staple of the Bedouin diet. White or yellow corn and rice were other dietary grains consumed frequently in the past. Meat appears to have been eaten during special occasions and to honor guests. Present-day Bedouin still rely heavily on bread and milk products. Lentils and chickpeas are common food items, as are seasonal vegetables and fruits, including onions, garlic, potatoes, tomatoes, and lettuce. Eggs are an important source of dietary protein for Bedouin families in the Bekaa today.

The Bekaa Valley has been central to the seasonal pastoral cycle of Bedouin tribes.[3] Historical accounts place Bedouin in the Bekaa as far back as the thirteenth century.[4] The Bekaa is an upland valley situated between Mount Lebanon in the west and the Anti-Lebanon Mountains in the east. The Litani River—the primary drainage of the Bekaa—flows southward from the area near Baalbek, traversing Mount Lebanon's southern edge and discharging into the Mediterranean. The Litani River was dammed in 1957 to form Lake Qaraoun. The reservoir's water is mostly used to generate electricity, with a limited amount used to support irrigation. The Orontes River flows northward into Syria, draining the northern Bekaa plain. The two rivers are also fed by copious springs in the Bekaa. In terms of size, the Bekaa is about 177 kilometers long and 9.6 to 16 kilometers wide with an average elevation of 762 meters. Its middle section spreads out more than its two extremities. The term Bekaa is derived from the Arabic plural of *buqʾā*, meaning a basin or place of stagnant water. The climate is semiarid to continental with unpredictable rainfall and periodic drought. The northern Bekaa is very dry, becoming semidesert, with a much wetter area south of the Beirut-Damascus road. The northern end of the valley is primarily used as grazing land by the Bedouin. Further south is where the more fertile soil is used to support farming. The northern Bekaa receives an annual average rainfall of only 230 mm (9 in.) compared to 610 mm (24 in.) in the south-central portion. Dry farming has long been the norm in the Bekaa, with the exception of ancient centers of irrigation like Baalbek. However, by 1998 some 52.1 percent of the total cultivated land in the Bekaa Valley was irrigated[5] and by 2005 this number had climbed to 67 percent.[6]

The expansion of state-led agriculture, propelled by the need to feed growing urban populations, has had far-reaching impacts on nomadic Bedouin peoples. The French colonial policy in Greater Syria during the 1920s and 1930s—informed by their colonial experience in North Africa—focused on securing the territory to facilitate economic exploitation.[7] It is estimated that two-thirds of Syrian territory on both sides of the Euphrates is steppe that was mostly inhabited by nomads and seminomads of Arab origin as well as Kurdish and Circassian groups. Military pacification of the steppe was therefore essential from the colonizer's perspective. The French created two mounted camel companies to subjugate the Bedouin. Military control over Bedouin was established by 1930 and facilitated, in part, by recognition of Syria's eastern borders by Turkey in 1929 and by Iraq in 1930. Delineation of state boundaries curtailed the mobility of Bedouin peoples, which, in turn, made it more difficult for them to subvert state authority. Once French authorities established military supremacy over Bedouin, colonial focus shifted to population and economic "development." Colonial officials sought to increase the indigenous population and thereby increase the number of agricultural laborers. They did this by providing medical aid (so as to reduce infant mortality), encouraging Bedouin settlement, and accelerating immigration as well as housing assistance for refugees, particularly Christian refugees (including Assyrio-Chaldeans from Iraq, and Armenians and Syrian Christians from Turkey).[8] The French vigorously supported religious minorities in order to undermine the growing Arab nationalist movement. Christians constituted a slight majority (51.7 percent) of the population of Lebanon, which was itself created by the French Mandate authority in 1920. The country was formed by attaching previously Syrian territory of the Bekaa Valley in the east to Mount Lebanon in the west. The western territory was expanded to the coast, incorporating the cities of Tripoli, Beirut, Sidon, and Tyre. The rest of Syria was divided into five semiautonomous territories designed to bolster French power by exploiting sectarian divisions within the country.

In 1932, slightly over a decade after the new nation of Lebanon was formed, French colonial officials conducted a census—the results of which were later used to establish Lebanon's confessional system of government and citizenship. Most Bedouins were not registered in the census (which until today remains the last official census to be undertaken in Lebanon). The reasons for Bedouin exclusion from the population count are related to seasonal absence due to migration and to reluctance on the part of many tribes to cooperate with a French colonial government seen as illegitimate.[9] This initial exclusion set the stage for Bedouin political marginalization from the nation-state, which continues up until the present (see below). To make matters worse, the French sold off pastureland, used by Bedouin in the Bekaa Valley, to peasant farmers. This started a mass wave of settlement, as Bedouin tribes found themselves with less grazing land to support their livestock, which in turn prompted them to sell off their livestock and pursue other means of livelihood, mostly farming. This gradual settlement and assimilation process is as old as civilization itself, but it has also worked in reverse in the past. Civilizational collapse, if not triggered by nomadic invasions themselves, often created a power vacuum that benefited nomadic populations. Farmers sometimes abandoned their fields and took up mobile pastoralism for a variety of reasons, including the drying up of former oases used to support settled agricultural communities and a desire to escape centralized state authority.

Unlike other states, Lebanon did not legislatively force the settlement of nomadic Bedouin tribes. The recent historical process of Bedouin settlement in the Bekaa is less a matter of government policy and more the result of "push" and "pull" factors of political-economic change. The push factors are linked to diminishing pastures, which accompanied the privatization of land, the rapid expansion of agriculture, the solidification of national boundaries, and urban sprawl. The pull factors are inextricably linked to social push forces, which gave rise to a new set of economic interests and calculations. The most recent wave of settlement in the Bekaa is the direct result of technological innovations in transport brought about by the second industrial revolution.

A fundamental change to Bedouin pastoralism occurred in the 1960s, as camels, which had traditionally been used for transport, were replaced with pickup trucks. Dawn Chatty explains some of the reasons for the shift from camels to mechanized transport in the Bekaa Valley. First, there were new hazards associated with camel transport once roads were paved—specifically, camels' flat padded feet were adapted to traveling on sand and have little traction on slippery road surfaces. Second, because camels tend to forage over large areas, the spread of orchard cultivation in the Bekaa made it increasingly difficult to monitor camels to ensure that they do not damage fruit crops.[10] The mechanization of transport led to major reductions in the nomadic movements of Bedouins and greater peasantization and commodification of their social economy. Migrations that once took months to complete now took days. After 1965, a large number of households began to remain in the Bekaa Valley during the winter, hiring out their trucks and services to neighboring villages and towns.

As Bedouins became less mobile, they developed even closer economic ties to peasant society. Oral histories from the present study indicate that many households during the 1970s ceased their seasonal migratory movements to the Syrian Desert and began establishing permanent settlements on purchased parcels of land in the Bekaa. Most land was a joint purchase by members of a patrilineal descent group (brothers or patrilateral cousins). Although Bedouins purchased land in the mid to late 1960s and sometimes before, they did not begin building houses until the 1970s and 1980s, as many lacked the means to do so. Most of the land was purchased near the same rural villages where Bedouin families entered into grazing agreements with peasant landowners during the summer portion of their nomadic pastoral cycle. In 2000–2001, there were more than eighteen Bedouin villages, enclaves, and neighborhoods in the Bekaa, most of which are informal settlements not recognized or listed on official maps.

Bedouin who continued to rely on pastoralism after the early 1970s replaced their winter migrations to the Syrian Desert with shorter migrations to the Bekaa's northern caves located on the border with Syria. In lieu of the natural pastures of the Syrian desert-steppe, which Bedouins had traditionally relied upon to sustain their herds through the winter, pastoralists began to rely on purchased feed. The first sugar-beet mill in the Bekaa began production at this time. The availability of purchased feed allowed the Bekaa Bedouin to develop a more sedentary pattern in the first place. Feed was often purchased by the truckload, depending on herd size. In addition to sugar-beet pulp, pastoralists also purchased *tibn* (cut straw or hay), date palm byproducts, and other palms as feed. Sheep were fed three times per day in the winter. Prior to the availability of purchased feed, the winter season was a precarious time for pastoralists, as inadequate natural forage meant that herd animals often starved to death.

These industrial developments in animal feed and transportation modernized and monetized Bedouin pastoralism. Pastoralists began to rely increasingly on money to cover the costs of winter feed, vehicle-related expenses (fuel and maintenance), and grazing contracts with peasant land-owners during the summer harvest. Oral histories indicate that families incurred debt during the winter as they purchased livestock feed, soap, tea, sugar, rice, and clothing from peasant shopkeepers and sold sheep, dairy products, and wool in the spring to pay off their debts. Some pastoral households also began to augment pastoralism with farming in order to pay for costly animal feed. In such instances, pastoralists specified that sharecropping partnerships (one-half or three-fourths portion of the crop for themselves) and, less often, tenancy contracts, were entered into in order to grow food for livestock and not human consumption. Bedouin families also began to employ their children, particularly unmarried adolescent girls, in agricultural wage labor. These new economic activities were made possible by trucks as well as purchased animal feed and the reduced mobility they afforded Bedouins. At the same time, diversification was necessitated by these technological developments and the destabilizing structural changes they helped set in motion.

To determine the scale and timing of these changes to traditional pastoral livelihoods, I asked Bedouin women about the primary occupation of their parents. Through these indirect work histories, I was able to obtain reliable information on parental occupation of 224 women.[11] Historical occupational designations derived from work histories are organized by time periods that correspond to the birth cohorts of women's mothers. Figure 2.1 illustrates changes in the Bedouin economic structure through time. The primary occupation of the oldest cohort, born during the early part of the twentieth century between 1899 and 1933 (with 1925 being the average year of birth), was pastoralism, which constitutes 62.7 percent of parent couples. The gradual decrease in pastoralism is evident, as is the sharp rise in agricultural sharecropping among the 1944–1965 cohort. Sharecropping rose from 4.9 percent in 1934–1943 to 30.4 percent in the 1944–1965 period—an increase of 25.5 percent from the previous cohort. The average year of birth among women born in the 1944–1965 period is 1952. Women in this cohort were marrying and beginning family-building in the 1970s. This period is marked by the mechanization of transport, cessation of the traditional seasonal pastoral cycle, the purchase of land for settlement, and overall peasantization of the Bedouin economy.

By the 1970s, most households began purchasing land in the Bekaa for household construction. To cover the costs of land purchase and home construction, Bedouins sold some or all of their herds, which increased their reliance on agricultural sharecropping and wage labor. The proletarianization of the Bedouin economy is relatively recent. Among the 1944–1965

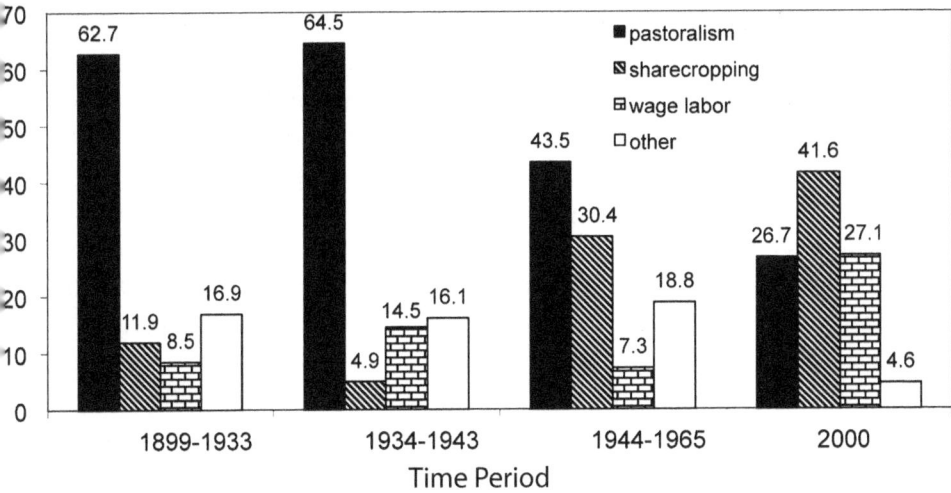

Figure 2.1. Bedouin women's parental occupation.

cohort, only 7.3 percent were employed in wage labor, compared to 27.1 percent at the time of the interviews in 2000 (see figure 2.1). The revolution in transportation facilitated the Bedouin sale of livestock to purchase land for residence, while the privatization of land as well as the delineation of state boundaries heralded the loss of traditional grazing lands. Accompanying these regional political-economic and ecological shifts were transformations in basic modes of social relations and social organization. The mechanization of transport (and the wave of capitalist development it both signified and induced) altered the interdependent grazing and trade relationship between village-dwelling agriculturalists and seminomadic Bedouin pastoralists. Reduced mobility afforded by trucks came with some serious drawbacks. As Bedouin became more sedentary and spent longer durations of time in the Bekaa, the question of where they would reside posed a problem. Bedouin families used to pitch their tents summer after summer on the farmland of peasant proprietors with whom they had entered into grazing agreements. The setting up of camp and grazing of flocks coincided with the harvesting calendar. Extended stays disrupted symbiotic partnerships. Disputes over crop damage became increasingly common. Bedouins are held responsible for damage done to peasant crops. Because Bedouin are cash-poor, they usually sacrifice a male sheep or provide other goods and services as compensation for crop damage. One of my Bedouin interlocutors described a grazing incident in which a landowner called the police and had to be appeased with "gifts."

Class distinctions between Bedouins and peasants were more firmly drawn as Bedouins became alienated from their grazing lands and livestock and more dependent on sedentary farming (sharecropping), wage labor (mostly agricultural), the underground economy, and, above all, money. The Bedouin sale of sheep and goat herds to finance the costs of fixed settlements accelerated peasantization and proletarianization. As a result, many Bedouins were left with only their labor to sell. The increasing reliance on fertilizers purchased on the market also reduced peasant reliance on Bedouin herds as a source of manure-fertilizer, further undermining the interdependency between the two parties and paving the way toward more unequal relations.

The general economic trend over the course of the last half century is one of decline in pastoralism and increase in sharecropping and agricultural/manufacturing wage labor. The historical recency of this profound economic shift from pastoralist to (landless) peasant and from pastoralist to proletariat demonstrates that for most Bedouin women aged forty years and over at the time of my fieldwork in 2000, tribal pastoral nomadism had been central to their lived experience. Regardless of their current occupation or trade in 2000, the majority of forty-year-olds and previous generations had, by that point in time, lived out at least half of their lives in a nomadic existence.

Historical Overview of Bedouin Fertility

Parallel to the historical transformations of traditional economic pastoralism and settlement structures were changes to women's fertility. Bedouin fertility has been subject to political-economic fluctuations associated with the broader process of demographic transition. The total fertility rate (TFR) can be calculated as either a cohort or period rate. As a cohort measure, it can be computed as the mean number of offspring ever-born to women of postreproductive age, in which case the TFR is a retrospective measure of cohort fertility. Fertility can also be computed as a cross-sectional (period) measure by summing the population's current age-specific fertility rates. If mortality is selective with respect to fertility (that is, if reproduction itself exposes the mother to an elevated risk of death), then retrospective TFRs may be biased downward, simply because women with low fertility have a better chance of surviving long enough to be interviewed.[12] Period and cohort TFRs are expected to be the same only if fertility rates have not changed over time. A comparison of period and cohort fertility rates among the Bekaa Bedouin suggests recent fertility change. The total-cohort fertility rate (TCFR) for Bedouin women born between 1942 and 1960 is 9.08 (see below), whereas the total-period fertility rate (TPFR) of Bedouin women calculated in 2000 is 6.55—an indication of recent fertility decline in the younger population.

The question of what constitutes high fertility is crucial, given that the small nuclear family (with fertility at or below replacement level) is not transhistorical but a recent feature of post-transitional societies. Bioanthropologists Kenneth Campbell and James Wood compiled cross-cultural data on total fertility rates (TFRs) from seventy pretransitional populations and found that 90 percent of human populations have total fertility rates (TFRs) between four and eight. Only three out of seventy populations (4.3 percent) in the sample have TFRs above 8.0, which are considered very high.[13] Using Campbell and Wood's criteria, older postreproductive or near-postreproductive Bedouin women with a completed family size of 9.08 can be considered to have very high fertility. Because earlier historical estimates of Bekaa Bedouin fertility are not available, I use indirect estimates to provide a window into past fertility. To derive historical measures of Bedouin fertility, I used a technique formalized by biological anthropologists Henry Harpending and Patricia Draper, referred to as the "frequency of family sizes."[14] The technique allows for estimation of fertility in the generation of the parents of a set of informants. I asked women informants whose mothers were postreproductive either at the time of the interview or at the time of their death: "how many live births did your mother have?" Women had no difficulty recounting their mothers' number of live births. Since women from larger families with more siblings are more likely to be accounted for than women from smaller families with fewer siblings, responses have to be weighted. Harpending and Draper have devised a method for weighting each observation so that a weight of one is assigned to those with one child, a weight of one-half to those with two children, and so on.

Table 2.1 provides observed and weighted frequencies of family sizes by birth cohort. I computed standard errors using the formula provided by Harpending and Draper.[15] The average family size of mothers who had at least one birth in the older cohort is 6.8 ± .30, compared to 8.3 ± .40 in the younger cohort. Older mothers in the early twentieth century born in the period 1899–1933 had an average year of birth of 1925. Mothers in the younger cohort who were born in 1934–1943 had an average year of birth of 1938. These data allow us to address the question of how long Bedouin fertility has remained at the upper end of the range of variation. Historical estimates of past fertility show that Bedouin women in the oldest cohort (1899–1933) have high fertility that is within the range of fertility variation reported by Campbell and Wood for pretransitional societies.[16] Very high

Table 2.1. Observed and weighted completed family size distributions of the mothers of informants by birth cohort

Family Size	Mothers Born 1899–1933		Mothers Born 1934–1943	
	Observed No.	Weighted No.	Observed No.	Weighted No.
1	0	0	0	0
2	1	0.5	1	0.5
3	1	0.33	0	0
4	5	1.25	1	0.25
5	6	1.2	2	0.4
6	6	1	6	1
7	9	1.29	7	0.86
8	9	1.13	7	0.88
9	6	0.67	9	1
10	7	0.7	14	1.4
11	3	0.27	4	0.46
12	4	0.33	5	0.43
13	1	0.08	2	0.15
14	2	0.14	0	0
15	1	0.07	1	0.07
16	0	0	2	0.13
17	0	0	0	0
18	0	0	1	0.06

fertility at the upper end of the range of variation for pretransitional societies is found among the younger cohort of Bedouin women (1934–1943). The fertility estimate for the 1934–1943 cohort (8.3) is similar to the direct estimate obtained for Bedouin women born over the period 1942–1960 (with an average year of birth of 1953). The parity distribution of 102 postreproductive or near-postreproductive women born in the 1942–1960 period is provided in table 2.2. The mean parity of Bedouin women born between 1942 and 1960 is 9.08. Completed family sizes range from zero to eighteen (see table 2.2). The indirect parity distributions of the 1934–1943 cohort are similar to the direct parity distributions of Bedouin women born between 1942 and 1960. Both the direct parity distributions shown in table 2.2 and the indirect parity distribution of women in the early past (1934–1943) shown in table 2.1 have a similar peak at parity 10. In contrast, there is a higher frequency of smaller sibships in the oldest cohort (1899–1933) shown in table 2.1.

Table 2.2. Completed family sizes of 102 postreproductive Bedouin women born 1942–1960

Parity/Completed Family Size

Parity	0	1	2	3	4	5	6	7	8	9	10	11	12	13	14	15	16	17	18	Total Women	Mean Parity	Median Parity
Observed No.	1	0	1	2	3	6	2	9	11	17	24	13	4	3	4	0	1	0	1	102	9.1	9

Taken together, direct and indirect estimates of Bedouin fertility show that the oldest cohort of Bedouin women born during the early Mandate years (1925 on average) and starting their family-building at the end of the Mandate period and early independence period already had high fertility, at 6.8 live births per woman on average. These women born during the early twentieth century had high, as opposed to very high, fertility. Fertility increased in the modern post-independence period as Bedouins made the transition to a more settled, peasant lifestyle. Historical estimates show that very high fertility is found among women born between 1934 and 1960. This means that very high fertility extends back to the cohort of women born at the end of the French Mandate period. These women were marrying and beginning their childbearing between the 1960s and 1980s—a period that coincides with the peasantization, modernization, and settlement of nomadic Bedouin in the Bekaa. Fertility remained high for five decades post-independence and then began to drop, initiating the modern decline in Bedouin fertility.

The period fertility rate of Bedouin women in 2000 is nearly 30 percent lower than the completed family size of older postreproductive women (for further discussion of Bedouin fertility transition, see chapter 6). A comparison of Bedouin period fertility and cohort fertility is provided in table 2.3. Table 2.3 indicates that postreproductive women, based on their ages in 2000, have higher age-specific fertility rates than women under forty years of age. Although the period measure is a synthetic indicator of fertility at one point in time among women of ages fifteen to forty-four, these younger women display lower fertility rates than the older cohort of women did when they were at the same age. The younger (synthetic) cohort of women also display a distinct fertility curve, with peak fertility occurring at ages twenty to twenty-four, as opposed to a peak at ages twenty-five to twenty-nine, seen in the older postreproductive cohort aged forty-five to fifty-four years in 2000.

The recent decline in Bedouin fertility has proceeded in tandem with the even sharper decline in desired family size. When asked about their family-

Table 2.3. Comparison of Bedouin period and cohort fertility

TPFR (Women aged 15 to 44 in 2000)			TCFR (Women aged 45 to 54 in 2000)		
Age Group	No.	Age-Specific Fertility	Age Group	No.	Age-Specific Fertility
15–19	13	.31	15–19	42	.16
20–24	29	.34	20–24	42	.34
25–29	43	.26	25–29	42	.49
30–34	55	.13	30–34	42	.36
35–39	39	.18	35–39	42	.30
40–44	23	.09	40–44	42	.11
Total	202	1.31	Total	42	1.76

Note: TPFR = $1.31 \times 5 = 6.55$
TCFR = $1.76 \times 5 = 8.80$

size preferences during reproductive-history interviews, women ages forty and over in 2000 indicated a preference for large families, with a mean desired family size of 8.02, and a modal desired family size of 10. In contrast, women under forty years of age in 2000 indicated a desire for much smaller families. The mean and modal desired family sizes among women under forty in 2000 were 4.98 and 4, respectively. These family-size preferences closely coincide with women's actual cohort fertility rates, although younger women's family-size preferences have dropped more sharply than their actual fertility rates.

In the midst of profound changes to Bedouin demographic and economic life, it is difficult for the casual observer to recognize that some important demographic continuities remain. Above all, there is considerable continuity in the patterning of marriage among the different age/birth cohorts of Bedouin women surveyed. In Bedouin society, reproduction occurs within the institution of marriage. The timing of marriage is remarkably stable among women forty and over in 2000 (born between 1942 and 1960) and women under forty in 2000 (born between 1961 and 1985). The mean and modal age at marriage is eighteen years in both cohorts. About half of the women in both age cohorts were married by the age of eighteen. In the older cohort, approximately 77.1 percent of women were married by the time they reached twenty years of age. In the younger cohort, 80.4 percent of women were married by the age of twenty. There is also historical continuity in terms of whom Bedouins marry. The proportion of women in the younger and older generations married to their first cousins is virtually unchanged— comprising almost two-fifths of all unions (see chapter 5). It is within these relatively stable parameters of marriage that we see some historical upward and later downward movement in fertility.

Bedouin fertility decline is part of an adjustment to economic adversity. The latter can be seen in the growing proportion of Bedouin families employed in wage labor, the broader downward trend of the national economy since the late 1980s, and the rising costs of modern sedentary life (in terms of childrearing, work-related expenses, housing, and transportation). Economic hardship has been invoked by many researchers to explain the decline of fertility in Arab countries. Eltigani Eltigani attributes economic struggles to the fact that most countries in the 1980s moved away from a public-sector- to a private-sector-dominated economy. Much of this economic restructuring was influenced by class interests in Arab countries and pressure from abroad, particularly multinational lending institutions, such as the World Bank and IMF.[17] Contrary to myths of high and unabating Arab fertility, the demographic transition in Arab countries is well under way. Fertility in eight Arab countries represented in the World Fertility Survey indicates a drop in the TFR from 6.5 in 1976–1981 to 4.0 in the 1990s. The decline in Arab fertility during this period was 38 percent, which was higher than the declines experienced in other world regions.[18] Bedouins are similarly adjusting their family sizes downward, although average fertility remains high, as opposed to very high, at this stage. At the same time that Bedouins in the Bekaa were adjusting their family sizes downward and becoming constituted as a landless and livestock-poor rural underclass, the country overall was experiencing political-economic and demographic transformation.

Regional and National Trends

The Bekaa Valley today is home to approximately 14 percent of Lebanon's 4–4.6 million inhabitants. At the time of my fieldwork, the population of the Bekaa was estimated at 539,448 with a population density of 129.6 people per square kilometer.[19] The Bekaa is also home to the highest concentration of Bedouin in Lebanon. The Bedouin live in the peripheral agricultural areas of the country. Their estimated population is 100,000–150,000, about 2.5 to 3 percent of the total national population.[20] Most Bedouins do not have Lebanese nationality and thus constitute de facto stateless persons, denied access to subsidized public health care, education, and employment opportunities. In 1958, Lebanon passed a law granting Bedouins who had not registered in the 1932 colonial census a distinctive "understudy" nationality status—a designation that recognizes the recipient's country of birth to be Lebanon. In 1994, the Hariri government granted, under the Nationalization Law of 1994, those individuals with "understudy" status from 1958 the right to Lebanese nationality. Nationality was only given to 10 percent of the Bedouin population in Lebanon.[21] This special nationality-status category still denies certain employment rights to its carriers, including the right to practice law. And there is yet another catch. The Bedouin who were given nationality cannot pass it on to their children, because it was granted to men and women as bachelors and spinsters, respectively, and not as married persons. This limited and contingent bestowal of citizenship is itself being challenged. As of 2000, the Lebanese Maronite League has appealed the Nationalization Law of 1994, arguing that it undermines Lebanon's sectarian stability. As a result of this appeal, the actual implementation of the 1994 law has been stalled, leaving the citizenship status of tens of thousands of Bedouins in limbo.[22]

Bedouin Arabs (most of whom are Sunni Muslims) constitute a marginalized minority in the Bekaa. The Bekaa region is a demographically composite place comprised mainly of Lebanese Arabs (Muslim, Christian, and Druze); but it is also home to a large minority of Palestinian Arab refugees (Muslim and Christian) and several ethnolinguistic minorities—the largest of which are the Christian Armenians. Some of the region's other residents include Syrian Arabs, Kurds (the second-largest ethnolinguistic minority in Lebanon), Turkmen, Gypsies, and mostly female Asian and East Asian domestic workers. The (Arab) ethnic and political makeup of the Bekaa could change in the near future due to the growing number of refugees entering the country. Lebanon has received more than ten thousand Iraqis fleeing the post-2003 U.S. invasion[23] and tens of thousands of Syrian nationals fleeing the political unrest in their country.[24] The Bekaa is one of Lebanon's six administrative governorates, or districts. The distribution of Lebanon's population across the six regional administrative governorates is as follows: Beirut (32.5 percent), Mount Lebanon (15.1 percent), North Lebanon (20.1 percent), South Lebanon (11.8 percent), Nabatiyeh (6.9 percent), and Bekaa (13.6 percent).[25] Around 88 percent of Lebanon's four-million-plus inhabitants reside in urban areas. The Bekaa Valley stands out as a rural farming region in an otherwise urbanized country. Directly related to urbanization is the declining percentage of the national population employed in agriculture—an economic trend of relatively recent historical origin.

One of the most significant changes in Lebanon's economy from independence to the present time has been the dramatic decline in the agricultural sector and the rise of a service economy. The Lebanese labor force continued to rely heavily on the agricultural sector up until the early 1970s. In 1967, it was estimated that 49 percent of the labor force in Lebanon relied on agriculture. Estimates from the early 1970s indicate a sharp decline, with one-fifth (20 percent) of the labor force in Lebanon deriving their livelihood from agriculture. By 1981, 9.2 percent of the total active population was employed in agriculture.[26] Two decades later (at the time of my fieldwork in 2000), the percentage of the labor force in Lebanon broke down as follows: 9 percent in agriculture, 11.2 percent in construction, 14.7 percent in industry, 22.3 percent in commerce, and 42.8 percent in services.[27]

Lebanon is primarily a service-oriented economy with a weak agricultural sector, but regional variation persists. The Bekaa is Lebanon's major agricultural area, extensively farmed for cereals (wheat, barley, and corn), vegetables (tomatoes, cucumbers, potatoes, and onions), fruit tree orchards (mostly citrus and pome fruits such as oranges, lemons, mandarins, apples, grapes, bananas, and peaches), and legumes (green beans, chickpeas, kidney beans, and green fava beans). During the war years, especially the 1980s, the Bekaa produced substantial amounts of hashish and opium. The Bekaa region comprises about 38–42 percent of the country's total agricultural land—the largest share of Lebanon's governorates. The distribution of the Bekaa Valley's harvested crop area (both rain-fed and irrigated production) in 2005 consisted of cereals (36.7 percent), fruit trees (26 percent), vegetables (22.5 percent), legumes (4 percent), olives (2.8 percent), agro-industrial crops (2.6 percent), other trees (0.6 percent), and other crops (4.8 percent).[28] Approximately 20.4 percent of the Bekaa's labor force—more than double the national estimate—continues to rely on agriculture for their livelihood.[29] In parts of the Bekaa Valley (Baalbek and Hermel) and the heavily war-affected rural areas of south Lebanon, agriculture comprises as much as 80 percent of local GDP and is the main source of employment and income.[30]

The sharp historical decline in the proportion of the total Lebanese workforce involved in agriculture and rapid urbanization in the country have occurred in connection with the rise of a service and remittance economy. Prior to the Civil War, between 1955 and 1975, capital in the form of bank deposits and trusts from the Gulf oil states and other countries in the region contributed to the rapid development of Lebanon. Tourism was also substantial prior to 1975, with more than one million visitors making their way to Lebanon each year.[31] Banking, education, and medical facilities, trade and transportation, tourism, and other service sectors fueled the rapid urbanization of Beirut and nearby Mount Lebanon. The rapid urbanization of the country after 1975 is also linked to massive rural exodus from disadvantaged areas in the Bekaa and the south, generated in large part by rural inhabitants trying to escape poverty and war-torn areas. Since the outbreak of the Civil War in 1975 and the loss in the value of the Lebanese currency during the 1980s—precipitated by the full-scale Israeli invasion of Lebanon in 1982—emigrants' remittances have become the backbone of the Lebanese economy. While to some extent Lebanon has been reliant on remittances since the first wave of immigration dating back to the nineteenth century, by the early 1980s remittances constituted about 50 percent of GDP. At the time of my return visit in 2007, Lebanon ranked eighth among the top ten remittance recipients in the world, receiving US$5.2 billion as remittances and $2.6 billion as Foreign Direct Investments.[32]

Massive out-migration and remittances have profound impacts on the economies of source communities. Since 1975, close to 1.3 million people—mainly professional and skilled workers—have left the country. The Bedouin were largely excluded from this external migration, because without Lebanese nationality they were unable to procure the required documents for travel. Extensive emigration has created a skewed population pyramid with a high female-to-male ratio in the country. Most emigrants consist of young males in the twenty- to twenty-five-year age group.[33] Large-scale Christian emigration, coupled with their lower fertility rate at home, altered the religious composition of the country. As of the early 2000s, 54 percent of people in Lebanon are Muslim, of which 32 percent are Shi'i, 21 percent Sunni, and 1 percent Alawi; 39 percent are Christian, of which 26.5 percent are Catholic (20 percent Maronite and 4.5 percent Greek Catholic or Melkite), 12 percent Orthodox (6 percent Greek Orthodox and 5 percent Armenian Apostolic), and 0.5 percent Protestant; and 7 percent are Druze.[34]

Many villages in rural Lebanon were emptied of their young workforce, as a result of both internal migration and emigration to foreign countries.[35] Such out-migration appears to have left a void in the rural economy, which the Bekaa Bedouin, particularly adolescent girls, were able to fill. Remittances also allowed some peasants to buy plots from landlords, which led to a surge in land speculation. The large depreciation of the Lebanese pound, together with the influx of diaspora remittances, led to expanded investment in land property (including rental land), which undermined the position of landlords, who had to sell a large part of their inherited lands to maintain their social status. The influence of the traditional feudal families or landlords had already been in decline from the mid-twentieth century, largely due to the growing influence of the financial sector, commercial groups, and other economic service sectors. While landowners were still a dominant class, particularly in rural areas, they no longer enjoyed the monopoly of power they once had.[36]

The rise of a new class of industrialists, bankers, and businesspeople changed the socioeconomic makeup of Lebanon. The absence of an effective public sector and the dominance of private capital—dramatically seen in late prime minister and billionaire Rafiq Hariri's "Solidere" company (founded in 1994) that took charge of Beirut's reconstruction in hopes of attracting Gulf, American, and European capital—have only exacerbated economic instability and imbalance in the country. In 1992, the Council for Development and Reconstruction (CDR) put forth a new thirteen-year plan (1995–2007) for public and social infrastructure reconstruction of Lebanon called Horizon 2000. Heavy borrowing as part of the plan has resulted in the explosion of public debt, from US$2 billion in 1992 to $15 billion in 1998 and to $38 billion in 2004.[37] Lebanon is a mineral-resource-poor country heavily dependent on external aid and remittances.

Income inequalities in Lebanon are considerable. It is estimated that nearly 8 percent of the Lebanese population (three hundred thousand individuals) live under conditions of extreme poverty and are unable to meet their most basic food and nonfood needs.[38] The richest 10 percent of families receive 35 percent of national income; the next 10 percent of middle-income families receive 15 percent of national income; and the poorest 80 percent (low-income families) receive 50 percent of national income.[39] Widespread high inflation between the mid-1980s and 1992 led to the deterioration of real incomes of Lebanese families.[40] Unbalanced economic development, war, and poverty-induced migration from all Lebanese rural areas, especially south Lebanon and the Bekaa Valley, have given rise to a proletarianized rural peasantry and a large urban proletariat in Greater Beirut. As Massoud Daher states, "In spite of its sectarian face, Lebanon is a country of enormous disparities between social classes and regional divisions."[41] The question is: can we frame and analyze Bedouin sociodemographic realities in terms of the same hierarchical class structures that order the lives of other Lebanese families?

3

(Un)Stratified Reproduction

Class, Tribe, and Culture

It is difficult to make unequivocal statements about the causes of demographic inequities, but it has become a social-science orthodoxy to assert that demographic disparities between rich and poor segments of society are widespread, with poor peoples being more likely to fall ill and die than more affluent groups. The main caveat is that most of the empirical support for socioeconomic disparities in health is based on macro North-South and between-country disparities.[1] Less is actually known about demographic and health disparities between local class or occupational groups within most countries and if/how those micro-level disparities have changed over time. The concept of "stratified reproduction"[2] has been developed to highlight how reproduction—the bearing, raising, and socialization of children throughout the life course—is differentially experienced along lines of social class and other axes of inequality. In this chapter, I present demographic and ethnographic evidence that verifies the presence of a wide class gap between Bedouin and peasant peoples in the region, but repudiates the presence of a wide occupational gap within Bedouin society. Because social class is communicated materially and morally, the cultural contours of class will be examined alongside the demographic and economic. My analysis of class, occupation, and tribe, as reflected through practice and values, is based on participant observation in Bedouin and peasant village communities in the Bekaa region. The boundary between being an anthropologist of the Bedouin and the daughter-in-law of a peasant family began to blur as I came to terms with my ethnographic engagement in both worlds.

Bedouins and Peasants: Class Relations and Cultural Differences

Upon the first week of my arrival in the Bekaa in 2000, a young peasant woman from my former husband's village pulled me aside and said, "I should tell you something . . ." She paused in mid-sentence with a serious look of concern on her face, as if to emphasize that she was about to reveal a devastating secret. "You know, we [fellahin] do not like them [Bedouin]." Her statement is emblematic of wider peasant antipathy toward the Bedouin. Eager to lend credibility to her allegations of Bedouin wrongdoing, she recounted numerous tales that were difficult to verify and (inadvertently) conveyed the opposite message of the one intended. She once told me about how a family friend of theirs—a wealthy landowner and small-scale agro-industrialist (he owns a chicken factory)—was having problems with his Bedouin employees. An alleged dispute had escalated to the point where both sides came armed with shotguns to resolve the matter. And this was only the beginning, as further peasant attempts to denigrate the Bedouin would soon follow. On one of the days I returned to my then in-laws' home with freshly baked bread prepared by one of my Bedouin interlocutors, a peasant neighbor came to visit. She was the same neighbor who remarked that I was spending too much time with the Bedouin and that I smelled like sheep. She walked into the kitchen, where my former mother-in-law and I were having bread with olives and labneh. "Who baked this bread?" she asked as she tore a small piece and gestured toward me. The response was not to her liking. With a disapproving look on her face, she smelled the bread and put it back down on the kitchen counter, stating that she could not eat unclean food.

Peasant remarks about unsanitary, unhygienic, and "dark" Bedouin bodies are commonplace and serve to racialize Bedouin Arabs as distinct from and inferior to non-Bedouin Arabs. Cleanliness also has religious connotations in that Muslims are required to ritually cleanse themselves before prayer. Peasants frequently allege that Bedouin men who come to pray at the mosque are "dirty," wearing shoes covered in mud. Non-Bedouin Arabs fault the Bedouin for their lack of devotion to daily prayer in general. Bedouin tattoos serve as another visible physical marker of religious blasphemy. Tattooing was a common cultural practice among Bedouin tribes in both Syria and Lebanon. Among Lebanese Bedouin, tattooing appears to have had symbolic significance as a marker of intertribal differences and as a form of cultural adornment (particularly facial tattoos, which young unmarried Bedouin women had done by Gypsy women).

Hand tattooing is sometimes undertaken by women and men as a medical treatment for joint or arthritic pain. Older Bedouin women still bear facial tattoos and both older men and women have tattoos on their arms or hands.[3] However, tattooing is prohibited in the Qur'an and serves to reinforce Bedouin religious unorthodoxy. Younger Bedouin women and men have discontinued the practice.

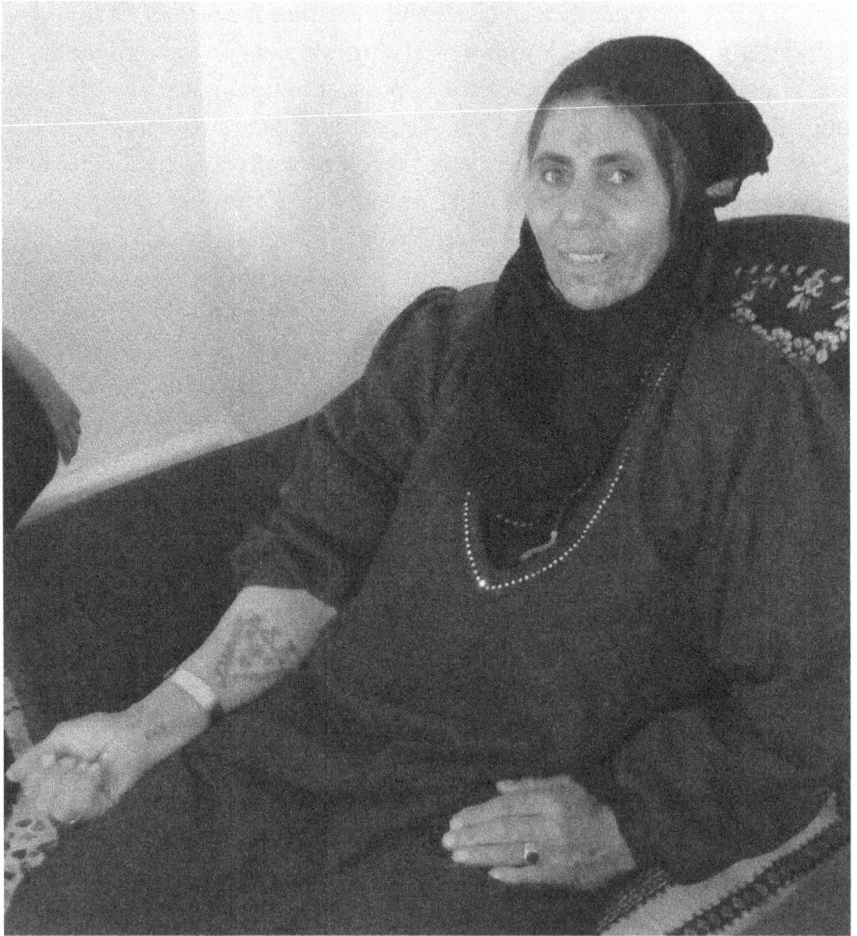

Figure 3.1. Bedouin woman with forearm and facial tattoos.

In addition to being scorned by peasants for their religious laxity or "primitive" tribal practices believed to be incompatible with Islam, other cultural cleavages figure prominently in peasant discourse. Bedouins are frequently described as "liars not to be trusted" and "difficult to under-stand." While the former establishes the Bedouin as morally and reputation-ally suspect, the latter differentiates the Bedouin on the basis of their dialect, which differs from colloquial Lebanese dialects. Bedouin personal names, especially those of women, are an important linguistic marker of Bedouin difference, which peasants use to brand Bedouins as different and "infe-rior." One Bedouin woman named her daughter ḥarba (She-war) because her daughter's birth coincided with the 1982 Israeli invasion of Lebanon. Another Bedouin mother chose to name her daughter Rḥayla (She-nomad) from the Arabic root *r-ḥ-l*, which means "to migrate or move." As recounted by Rḥayla herself, on the day she was born, spring was nearing its close and family members within her mother's camping unit were planning to migrate. "My mother said to them, 'I cannot move today; I am about to give birth.'" But forage for their flocks was scarce and so family members continued packing up their tents and other belongings, leaving the expectant mother with two women to assist her in her delivery. After giving birth, Rḥayla's mother, accompanied by the two women, eventually caught up with their party. "When they saw my mother, they asked, 'What did you have, a boy or a girl?' My mother replied, 'I had a girl.' 'What did you name her?' 'I named her Rḥayla.'" In naming children, Bedouin mothers will often draw upon salient memories or events surrounding that child's birth.

Pejorative, racialized, and classist discourses on Bedouin are dominant in peasant society, although they are sometimes concealed by patron-client relations.[4] I do not wish to imply that classist peasant narratives on Bedouin Arabs are never contested by peasants, only that I found alternative discourses to be uncommon. I do recall my mother-in-law at the time, a well-respected elder peasant woman in her own village community, proudly proclaiming, "I am a Bedouin woman." In asserting her social connectivity to the Bedouin, she told me how she used to work as an agricultural laborer, when she was still young and unwedded, alongside other unmarried peasant girls—in much the same way that Bedouin girls do today. Bedouin have increasingly assumed an economic role previously held by poor peasant women. When considering Bedouin-peasant class tensions from a Bedouin vantage point, the question becomes: how do Bedouin articulate their status vis-à-vis peasants?

A few of the Bedouin men and women I met possessed a keen class consciousness. One Bedouin man from the North Bekaa succinctly describes the exploitation of Bedouin by peasants as follows: "We do the hard work; they [peasants] profit . . . Bedouin men apply for jobs with the government and always get turned down. We are treated like sheep bred for sacrifice." Bedouin do not have the same employment opportunities as peasants, because most Bedouins lack citizenship. The class tensions between Bedouin and fellah are aptly described by Abu Barakāt, a Syrian Bedouin man who has been living and working in Lebanon for more than ten years:

> There is between them a perspective that each has for the other. There is a scornful regard that the villager possesses, be he fellah or Bedouin. If you ask any fellah, he will say, "Who is that piece of Bedouin? He is [barely] worth a franc." And if you ask a Bedouin, he will say that

the fellah is without roots. You see, the *na'ra* (feud) between them still exists. Even if you forget the Bedouin and the fellah and bring the Lebanese gentleman [this is true]. The Lebanese considers the Syrian to be nothing. This is especially true of [Lebanese] Christian peoples who see the Syrians who are present in Lebanon as nothing. The feud between them [the various groups] exists in religion and society; it exists between the Bedouin and the fellah, the Sunni and the Shʻi, the Muslim and the Christian, and the Syrian and the Lebanese.

Abu Barakāt eloquently frames Bedouin-peasant divisions within the broader context of Lebanese intra- and intersectarian as well as national tensions in the region. I expected to find ample Bedouin references such as these to class divisions, but instead I was surprised by how frequently I heard Bedouins insist that social differences between them and peasants were largely dissolving.

Women and men describe how, while they used to be nomadic Bedouin, they are now *Badu ḥaḍar* ("civilized"/modern/settled Bedouin). That is, they presently reside in villages, send their children to school, and read and study the Qur'an. Citizenship, land, running water, literacy, paved village roads, and jobs in government are all aspects of modern peasant life that are desired. However, not all features of peasant life are embraced. Bedouin acknowledge important cultural and moral differences linked to generosity, honor, modesty, and gender. Bedouin women and men frequently contrast Bedouin hospitality and generosity with that of peasants and find the latter wanting. A Bedouin man in his early forties describes the distinctiveness of the Bedouin code of politeness and generosity thus: "When you enter a Bedouin house, you realize that guests are treated in a distinct way. Guests are greeted and welcomed with respect, kindness, and generosity. The Bedouin is embarrassed in front of his guest. The fellah does not care."

The generosity and hospitality bestowed upon strangers is an extension of the generosity[5] accorded to relatives. The phrase "relatives of the heart" is sometimes used to describe emotional bonds between nonkin. It is difficult not to notice the hospitality and generosity accorded to guests. At a minimum, coffee is brewed for guests, often followed by the serving of heavily sweetened tea. Coffee rituals in particular help cement bread-and-salt friendship as well as kinship bonds between host/giver and guest/receiver. It is also not uncommon for hosts to prepare *ghada* (the afternoon meal) or even offer an honorary sacrifice of sheep to welcome a guest. Whether visitors are welcomed with coffee/tea, extended a lunch invitation, or honored with a slaughter of an animal depends on the context and relationship

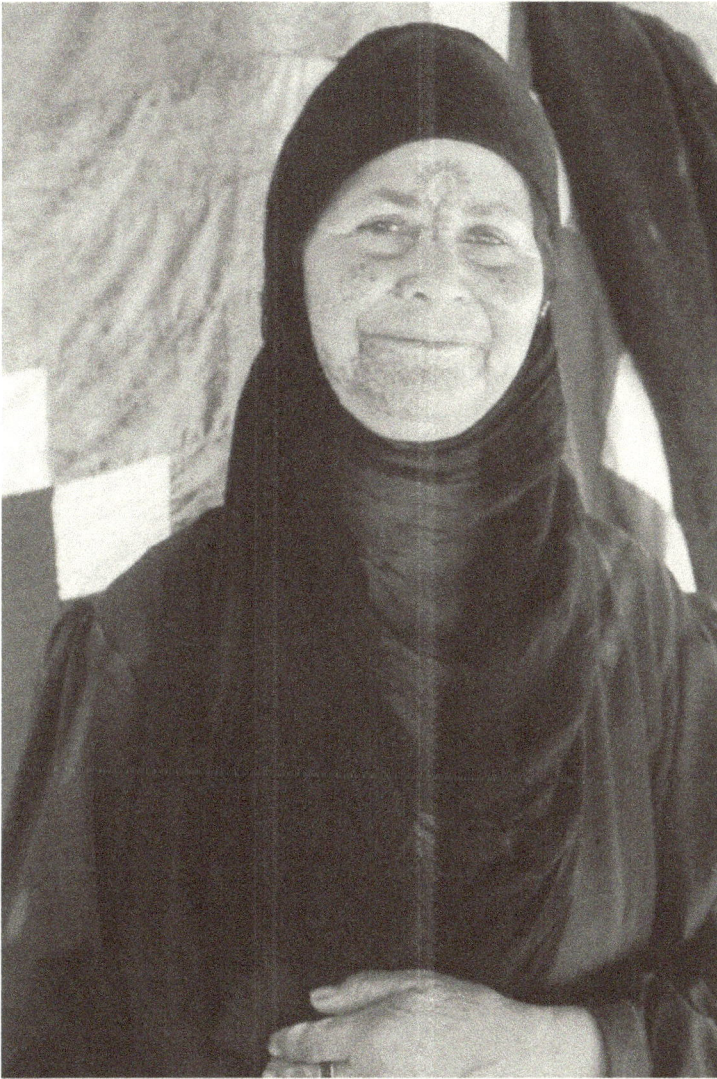

Figure 3.2. Syrian Bedouin woman welcoming visitors to her family's tent house. (We pulled up to their camp in the Syrian Desert, much to the dislike of her Saudi employer-shepherd, who followed us there and was determined to get rid of us. She warned me of our guide, whom she described as a "liar," which he was).

between host and guest as well as the status of the guest. On numerous occasions after an interview, I was sent off to my host family with milk, yogurt, freshly baked bread, and crates of vegetables—everything from cabbages to potatoes. The Bedouin are consummate hosts, and the artful style of their greeting is enough to flatter and warm the heart of the sternest and most cynical of visitors.

Bedouins also proudly assert their strong sense of modesty and virtue, finding fault with what they see as sexual impropriety on the part of both peasant men and women. Although rules of honor and modesty are applied more stringently to Bedouin women, there is still a strong societal expectation of sexual propriety on the part of Bedouin men. A Bedouin mother of eight, with whom I spent considerable time, describes the moral virtue of her six sons and Bedouin men in general:

> He [the Bedouin man] protects. *Bi-ḥāfiẓ ʿala l-ʿarḍ.* (He guards/protects/sustains honor.) There is no one more *sharīf* (honest/noble/upright) than the Bedouin son. You could stay with us for over ten years and they would not come near you [i.e., touch you]. They would protect your honor as they would their own sister's. They would treat you and care for you as a sister.

An older Bedouin couple spoke similarly of masculine honor: "We respect the honor of others. We respect the daughters of peasants and those of our own." The mother and father explained that Bedouin parents and elders, unlike peasant families, do not tolerate sexual promiscuity on the part of their sons. Indeed, male modesty is apparent in the number of affirmative

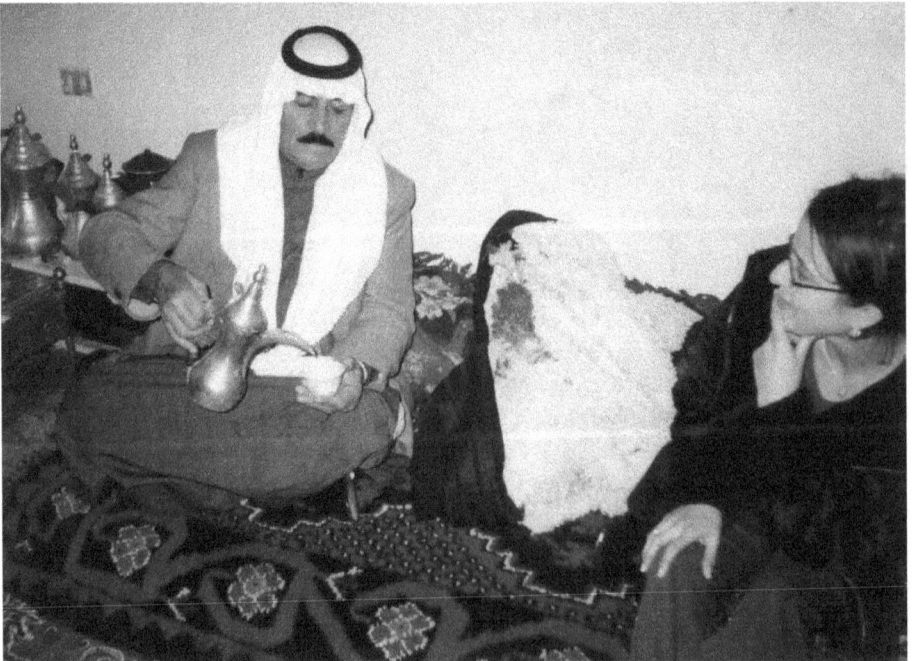

Figure 3.3. Bedouin tribal shaykh serving coffee to welcome guest (author).

responses we received to the query about whether men were virgins at the time of their first marriage. (A similar question was not posed to Bedouin women.)

Closely linked to self-ascribed distinctions of honor and modesty surrounding sexual conduct is the cited moral calculus underlying marriage decisions (see also chapter 5). In 2007, one of my Bedouin interlocutors married to his patriparallel cousin explained the importance of knowing the family of one's partner:

> There is a man who wanted to arrange his daughter's marriage. She is a dark-skinned girl and unsightly, with each tooth the size of a little finger. All the people [from the groom-to-be's family] would ask the [groom-to-be's] father, "Why are you going to marry off your son like this?" The father [of the groom-to-be] said to them, "Tomorrow, you will see. The family of the girl is good. I know her *aṣl* (lineage/descent/ancestry/origin). I know her father and her grandfather, *musalsalita* (her sequence/succession/chain)." And [in time] she had a son who is *aṣīl* (wellborn). The people thought that she was going to have children who were crazy and dim-witted. But it turned out she had a son who is *aṣīl* just as the [groom's] father said. Today, men and women care more about looks and beauty not *aṣl*. They do not ask about her [the bride's] family. They get married without knowing the family of the girl.

Bedouins pride themselves on the attention given to family lineage in selecting a marriage partner. Past family history provides a window into the future—an index of a potential marriage partner's moral reputation and ability to produce viable healthy offspring. My interlocutor laments the failure of peasantized Bedouins in the Bekaa today to live up to ancestral Bedouin rules of conduct. Marriage is central to the constitution of the self and becomes the site of moral degeneration. Modern Bedouins who fail to observe customary marriage practices are faulted for becoming peasantlike.

But perhaps the most important difference between Bedouin and fellah is the distinct cultural heritage of Bedouin tribal nomadism itself. The Bedouin tell their children stories of pastoral lives lived on foot, where camels were used to transport tents and nomadic movements followed the seasons. They tell of how tribes united in the Syrian Desert in the springtime, how they shunned military conscription, and how, when crossing national borders, they required no forms of identification issued by the state. Thus, while the Bedouin see themselves as modern and modernizing members of society, their nomadic past remains an important source of identity and one of proud distinction. Bedouins do not see these distinctions as sources of conflict that preclude their participation in wider peasant society. While a distinct nomadic tribal and cultural heritage is part of their identity, the Bedouin have other parallel identities. The Bedouin recognize that their cultural emphasis on honor, though slightly different in form, is found in Arab societies in general. Above all, Bedouins have a strong sense of identity as Muslims. Bedouin women and men emphasized their membership in Lebanese state society as both Lebanese and Muslims. The Bedouin are less prone to acknowledge tensions or class conflict with peasants and repeatedly affirm, "We are all Muslims." While peasants seek to denigrate, shun, and question the Bedouin as liminal Muslims, the Bedouin posit their Muslim identity as a unifying and equalizing principle of social life.

The Economic and Demographic Markings of Bedouin-Peasant Class Differentiation

The socioeconomic markings of class have emerged in parallel with increased peasantization of the Bedouin economy. The economic basis of Bedouin-peasant differentiation is beyond dispute. The Bedouin of the Bekaa Valley are virtually landless—they do not own *productive* land. Table 3.1 summarizes land and livestock ownership status of Bedouin households in 2000–2001. Out of 240 women interviewed about their household land ownership, approximately 71.2 percent were found to be landless. The mean and median plot size among the 240 Bedouin interviewed in 2000–2001 are 3.5 and 0.0 dunums (SD = 16.95), respectively. Most Bedouin women stated during interviews that while they do not own productive land, they do own the land on which their house rests. Eighty percent of Bedouins live in permanent stone/cement houses. Yet, even here it was apparent that families do not possess secure tenure on their properties. Bedouin without citizenship have experienced great difficulties in buying land and building homes. Some peasants refused to sell them land. Many had to put land in

Table 3.1. Household ownership status of sheep/goats, cows, and land, 2000–2001

Animals/Land	Yes		No	
	No.	%	No.	%
Sheep and goats	104	43.3	136	56.7
Cows	26	10.8	214	89.2
Land	69	28.8	171	71.2

the names of relatives or friends (including peasants) with valid federally issued forms of identity. Several Bedouin men reported bribing government officials so that they could complete household construction in the absence of a permit. Much of Bedouin household construction took place at night in order to avert law enforcement authorities. Still, oral histories indicate that some Bedouin men were nonetheless arrested for "illegal" construction.

Of the remaining 28.8 percent of Bedouin households that own productive farmland, 60.9 percent own 3 dunums or less. The mean and median farm size among the sixty-nine Bedouin families who own land are 12.2 and 2.0 dunums (SD = 30.1), respectively. In addition to extreme land scarcity and parcelization, Bedouins are experiencing alienation from their herds of sheep and goats. More than half of Bedouins interviewed (56.7 percent) lack ownership of the means of production in the form of sheep and goats, and the vast majority (89.2 percent) do not own cows. In work histories, women recounted selling livestock in the 1970s and 1980s to buy land and build a house, which increased Bedouin reliance on agricultural sharecropping and wage labor. Tables 3.2, 3.3, and 3.4 provide information on the distribution of land, sheep/goats, and cows, respectively. Of the 104 Bedouin families who own livestock, the average holdings are 126.2 head of sheep, 24.5 head of goats, and 0.7 head of cows.

Estimates of peasant land holdings in the Bekaa Valley, Lebanon, give us a glimpse into the extent of the economic disparity between Bedouin and fellah. Daher estimates average land holdings in the Bekaa in 1963 at 2.6 hectares, or 26 dunums. At this time, roughly 50 percent of smallholders in the Bekaa owned 11 percent of total cultivated land.[6] Land fragmentation is part of a wider pattern in Lebanese society. A more recent study, from 1999—roughly the same time as work-history interviews were conducted

Table 3.2. Size of land holdings among households that own land, 2000–2001

Size of land (dunum)	No.	%
<1	12	17.4
1–9	40	58.0
10–29	9	13.0
30–49	2	2.9
50+	6	8.7
Total	69	100.0

Note: 1 dunum = .1 hectare.

Table 3.3. Household herd size of sheep/goats among households that own herds, 2000–2001

Number of Sheep and Goats	No.	%	% of Total Herd
1–9	15	14.4	.4
10–49	19	18.3	3.0
50–99	14	13.5	5.5
100–49	11	10.6	8.1
150–99	14	13.5	14.1
200–49	10	9.6	13.0
250–99	7	6.7	11.6
300–49	5	4.8	9.6
350–99	1	0.9	2.2
400–49	2	1.9	5.1
450+	6	5.8	27.4
Total	104	100.0	100.0

Table 3.4. Distribution of cows among households that own cows, 2000–2001

Number of Cows	Number of Households	%
1	4	15.4
2	6	23.1
3	1	3.8
4	2	7.7
5	3	11.5
6	1	3.8
7	2	7.7
8	1	3.8
10	2	7.7
15	1	3.8
25	1	3.8
30	1	3.8
50	1	3.8
210	26	100.0

with the Bedouin—shows that there are 35,146 agricultural holders in the Bekaa, with an average farm size of 29.3 dunums, more than double that found among Bedouin agricultural holders. The average farm size in Lebanon overall is 12.7 dunums,[7] which is four times higher than the Bedouin average of 3.5 dunums. Almost 75 percent of all farmers in Lebanon cultivate an area less than 10 dunums each and account for 20 percent of total cultivated land.[8] In terms of livestock, statistics from Lebanon's Ministry of Agriculture indicate that the Bekaa has 6,429 livestock holders (28 percent of the national total). Peasant herd owners average 43.4 head of sheep, 32.1 head of goats, and 3.3 head of cows.[9] Bedouin herd owners fall below the average livestock holdings of goats and cows in the Bekaa, but have approximately triple the average sheep holdings at 126.2 head. The Bedouin advantage in sheep ownership is somewhat countered by the fact that they have larger family sizes and more mouths to feed (see below). Peasant herd owners are also more likely to own land, which can be used to grow crops for livestock or human consumption.

In addition to Bedouin-peasant class disparities, class-specific demographic differentials are also apparent, with Bedouin having higher fertility and higher infant mortality. The Bedouin infant mortality rate in the Bekaa in 2000 was 53 per 1,000. In contrast, the infant mortality rate in Lebanon was almost half that found in Bedouin society, at 28 per 1,000 in 1986–1995, and it remained the same in 2002.[10] The infant mortality rate among peasant communities in the Bekaa Valley in 1986–1995 was 40 per 1,000[11]—a figure still lower than the 2000 estimate of Bedouin infant mortality. The Bedouin infant mortality rate is almost double that found in Lebanon overall.[12] National-level estimates of life expectancy further underscore social-class distinctions between rural Bedouin and the urban Lebanese population. Life expectancy in Lebanon—estimated between seventy-one and seventy-four years in 2000[13]—is approximately ten years higher than Bedouin life expectancy (see chapter 4 for a discussion of gender differences in early child mortality and estimates of life expectancy at birth).

Bedouin-peasant fertility differentials are even more pronounced. Bedouin women born between 1942 and 1960, who were postreproductive or near postreproductive at the time they were interviewed (see table 2.2), had a completed family size of 9.08 (SD = 2.86). The cohort fertility rate among peasant women in the Bekaa born between 1947 and 1951, who had virtually completed their childbearing at the time of a 1996 survey, was found to be 5.86.[14] A comparison with Bekaa Bedouin women born during the same five-year time period (n = 23 Bedouin women), reveals a substantially higher total-cohort fertility rate of 9.70—a difference of more than four live births. At the national level in Lebanon, fertility had already begun to decline in the 1970s. Estimates of Lebanese fertility around the time of my fieldwork in 2000 show urban Lebanese fertility to be far lower than Bedouin fertility in the Bekaa. The total-period fertility rate in Lebanon dropped from 3.2 in 1990 to 2.2 in 2000.[15] Between 1991 and 1995, the total-period fertility rate in Lebanon was 2.5. The most reliable recent estimates for Lebanon in 2006 show a continuing decline, with Lebanese fertility slightly below replacement level, at 1.95.[16] In the Bekaa Valley region, fertility is only slightly higher than the national average. The total-period fertility rate from 1992 to 1995 in the Bekaa was 2.7.[17] By comparison, even relying on period estimates of Bedouin fertility, Bedouin women give birth to four more children, on average, than their non-Bedouin Arab counterparts in the Bekaa.

The subordinate health status of Bedouin in relation to peasants is part and parcel of their class subordination in Lebanon. As a region overall, the Bekaa Valley faces some important health challenges, especially in terms of child health. The Bekaa has the highest rates of stunting and dehydration among children under five, the highest prevalence of cough among children six to eleven months, and the second-highest levels of infant mortality of Lebanon's six governorates.[18] Bedouin constitute marginalized rural communities in the Bekaa that generally lack access to government-subsidized medication or treatment distributed in dispensaries and clinics near their own villages and thus must seek medical care in either the nonprofit sector or in increasingly costly and unregulated private clinics.[19] Because most Bedouins do not have citizenship, they have difficulty tapping into government health-care services. The one important exception is the primary and secondary health care provided by nongovernmental organizations (NGOs). Since around the mid-twentieth century, humanitarian NGOs like the Lebanese Red Cross, the Lebanese Red Crescent, and the Palestine Red Crescent have provided health services in the region via permanent or semipermanent health centers and clinics that treat stateless and underprivileged groups. Peasant devaluation and discrimination against Bedouin is commonplace, however, and serves to obstruct their access to reproductive and child health services.

Bedouin-peasant class distinctions are part of a broader regional pattern. Health disparities like those found between Bedouin Arabs and non-Bedouin Arabs in Lebanon have been observed in the Middle East and North Africa. By the 1950s, Bedouins were among the worst off in Arab societies in terms of most indicators of socioeconomic status, with limited access to modern health care and having among the region's highest levels of infant mortality.[20] Donald Cole explains how class divisions are one of the consequences of colonialism, which disrupted kin-based pastoral production. Examples of colonial assault on Bedouin Arab peoples can be seen in Palestine, Algeria, Libya, Egypt, Syria, and Iraq. Algeria represents one of the more extreme examples owing to 132 years of French colonialism in which colonists appropriated the best land and facilitated the sale of land to European colonists via land privatization, pushing Bedouins and poor sedentary peasants onto marginal areas.[21]

High fertility and population growth rates in Bedouin communities today reinscribe Bedouin-peasant class divisions. In his essay "Demographic Regimes as Cultural Systems," Philip Kreager observes that once vital processes within cultural systems are established as a pattern, they "become objects of cultural interpretation, by which people identify themselves with particular groups, and contrast their behavior to others."[22] Anthropological demographers Jane and Peter Schneider have little difficulty applying Kreager's thesis to Sicilian classes in Mediterranean Europe. In Villamaura, Sicily, class formation sparked both demographic and moral difference within the community. When members of the upper classes were asked why high fertility persisted among the class of landless peasants, they responded with expressions that linked poverty to progeny and sex. One expression in particular lent itself to the title of the book: "sexual embrace is the festival of the poor."[23] The sexualization of poverty in Europe extends back to the founding of the science of population by Thomas Malthus at the end of the eighteenth century. Malthus argued that the poor classes were poor because of their sexual licentiousness and "early and improvident" marriages (see chapter 6). Class and class-specific demographic distinctions between Bedouin and fellah are articulated somewhat differently.

As mentioned previously, class tensions between Bedouin and fellah in the Bekaa are not usually culturally articulated in the idiom of poverty-sex-progeny, but in terms of racial uncleanliness, religious laxity, and linguistic difference. Pejorative comments about Bedouin "zeal" for childbearing were more often made by urban residents of Beirut with whom I spoke than rural residents of the Bekaa. (Urban elites have difficulty distinguishing Bedouins from Gypsies and are more likely to articulate Orientalist stereotypes, such as that of the lascivious Bedouin Arab man surrounded by his harem wives and, in the words of one student from an elite college in Beirut, "children whose names he cannot even remember.") There seems to be an underlying admiration of large families among village peasants, although the costs of raising children are seen as prohibitive of large families. There is even faint praise for men who father numerous children. A peasant father in his mid-twenties named 'Alī drew much attention after the birth of his third child, who was unplanned. His friends laughingly teased, "Haven't you heard of television? You need to watch TV or find something else to do." Having three children in a relatively short span of four years seemed to raise questions, but also provided a boost to 'Alī's virility.

While Bedouin childbearing may not always meet with direct disapproval, Bedouin are reproached for not attending to their children's education. Most postreproductive Bedouin women did not attend school; however, many families place their children in school up until fifth grade. After that point, children have to have their identity cards to remain enrolled, which is problematic for most Bedouins, who lack Lebanese citizenship. The costs of schooling are also prohibitive. A few families I met who had relatives in Syria or lived close to the Lebanese border with Syria reported placing their children in Syrian schools. For the most part, Bedouin families cannot afford private schools, and access to government schools is limited. Bedouin children who do attend school in Lebanon also face discrimination—both from peasant schoolteachers and student peers—making it an extremely difficult social environment in which to learn. The educational gap between Bedouins and fellahin provides fertile ground for class devaluation and tension. With the increased peasantization of Bedouin society, younger couples express a clear desire for smaller families, explaining that by having smaller families, they will be able to provide each child with an appropriate education, suitable clothing, and other comforts (see chapter 6 for further discussion of falling Bedouin fertility).

I have thus far characterized social-class relations and class-specific demographic disparities between Bedouins and peasants in the Bekaa Valley, Lebanon. The next sections take up questions of unstratified reproduction *within* Bedouin communities, focusing on economic and demographic structure at the local level.

Bedouin Economic Structure

Given the prevalence of landlessness in Bedouin communities in the Bekaa (with almost three-fourths of the population without land) and the miniscule holdings of those who own land—averaging less than one-half of a hectare (3.5 dunums, or 0.35 hectares)—most Bedouins seek employment as sharecroppers and wage laborers. Only a small portion of land in Lebanon is designated as public land. The vast majority of land in the Bekaa is privately owned by non-Bedouin Arabs, some of whom are absentee landowners. As a result, a minority of prosperous peasants own the means of production necessary for securing rental of grazing land for herds, agreements for sharecropping or tenancy, and for "hiring in" agricultural wage laborers. Because the employment activities of couples varied over the life course, Bedouin were classified according to the couples' dominant occupation since marriage. Work histories from the current study reveal that most Bedouins are involved in sharecropping (*sharika*) (41.6 percent), followed

by wage labor (*shughl bī l-faʿil or shughl bī l-ujra*) (27.1 percent), and pastoralism or shepherding (*shughl bī l-ṭarsh*) (26.7 percent). The remaining 4.6
percent work in miscellaneous rural trade occupations (e.g., milk collection,
butchering, rural crafts, truck driving/transport, small shopkeeping, and
petty trade).

Sharecropping as a mode of production was perceived by Karl Marx to
be a transitional arrangement between feudalism and capitalism. However,
Marx's conception has been refined, as sociologists and historians have since
demonstrated that sharecropping existed in social formations where neither
capitalism nor feudalism existed[24] and that it continues to exist side by side
with the capitalist mode of production.[25] The type of sharecropping found
among Bedouin households can be defined as an investment shared by the
landlord and tenant farmer, where the latter acts, mainly, as a passive partner.[26] The landlord provides the land and water, half of all the other inputs
(e.g., seedlings, fertilizers, and pesticides), while labor (harvesting, weeding, and so on) is solely provided by the tenant. Machinery is sometimes
provided by the landlord and sometimes rented. Each party receives half of
the net marketed yield. In terms of the division of labor under sharecropping, there is a great deal of cooperation among members of the household
and sometimes extended family. The gendered division of labor is such that
men normally do the plowing and harrowing, while other work is shared
between men and women. Women and children tend to do the weeding.
Labor assistance is sometimes provided by a woman's husband's brother and
his children. Tenant farming, wherein a tenant rents a plot of land for a short
duration, does not require a fifty-fifty split of the crop, but requires larger
capital outlays up front. Since only a small number of Bedouin families were
found to have engaged in tenant farming for a couple of years and usually
returned to sharecropping, tenant farmers and sharecroppers were placed
in the same occupational category.

Bedouin who work as wage laborers are mostly employed in agriculture
and work as daily laborers. The price of labor within the agricultural system is determined by the market. In 2000, workers received a daily wage
of 5,000 Lebanese pounds (approximately US$3.33). Those Bedouin em-
ployed in manufacturing mostly work in local agro-industries (chicken
and cheese factories), packaging companies, cement plants, or gas stations.
The gendered division of labor is more distinct within wage-earner families. Women wage laborers either help supplement the husband's income by
working alongside other female relatives (so as not to contravene gender
norms of honor and modesty) or stay at home and perform domestic work.
Married women do not normally work alongside their husbands in facto-

ries. Subsidiary or supplementary forms of production are common among wage laborers. The underground economy can provide extra income for struggling wage laborers. One woman, in recounting her and her husband's economic activities in the underground economy (fuel oil smuggling), paused to take in their home and its furnishings, before saying, "Ḥabibtī (my dearest), work in wage labor does not build a house."

Pastoralism as practiced by Bedouin in the Bekaa Valley today is characterized by private ownership of livestock (sheep and goats) with heavy reliance on rented grazing land and purchased feedstuffs. Bedouin pastoralists largely acquire livestock through inheritance and, sometimes, through purchase from the market. There are historical examples of shareherding contracts. Partner contracts are normally two to five years in duration. Bedouin provide the labor and peasant herding partners provide the sheep, which are evenly divided at the end of the contract period. However, such contracts were a rarity at the time of work-history interviews in 2000. Most Bedouins are independent pastoralists, relying predominantly on family labor for herding. Indirect work histories indicate that some households relied on hired Syrian Bedouin labor at the beginning of the family life cycle, when couples did not yet have children or their children were too young to work. Hence, the use of Syrian hired shepherds is mostly associated with the older parental generation born between 1899 and 1943. A Bedouin woman in her early forties, whose parents possessed substantial livestock holdings, explained that her parents preferred to hire Syrian, not Lebanese, Bedouin, because Syrian Bedouin slept alone in the *sahel* (open plain) and "had no fear of wolves." In terms of ownership of the means of production, it is almost invariably the case that livestock are privately owned. There are plenty of cases of joint herding on the part of brothers and other close agnates, but each party retains their share if/when they split up.

The sexual division of labor among pastoralists reflects interdependency and complementarity between husband and wife. Men are usually responsible for grazing the livestock, purchasing feed, and transporting livestock. Bedouin women (and children) are responsible for setting up the tent, collecting firewood, roping the herds and milking them twice daily, and preparing butter, yogurt, and cheese for household consumption. It is not uncommon for adult women and children to graze flocks. Bedouins will also sometimes rely on extended family members, particularly a man's brother's sons, to assist in grazing. Bedouin pastoralists today largely rely on the income derived from the daily sale of milk to dairy companies, which purchase milk by the kilogram. At the time of the interviews in 2000–2001, a kilogram of milk was priced between five hundred and seven hundred Leba-

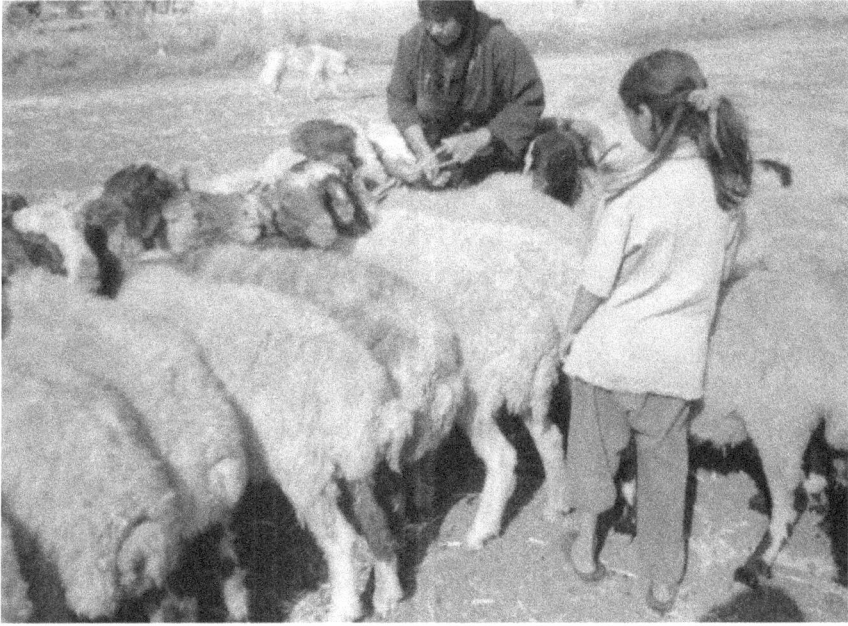

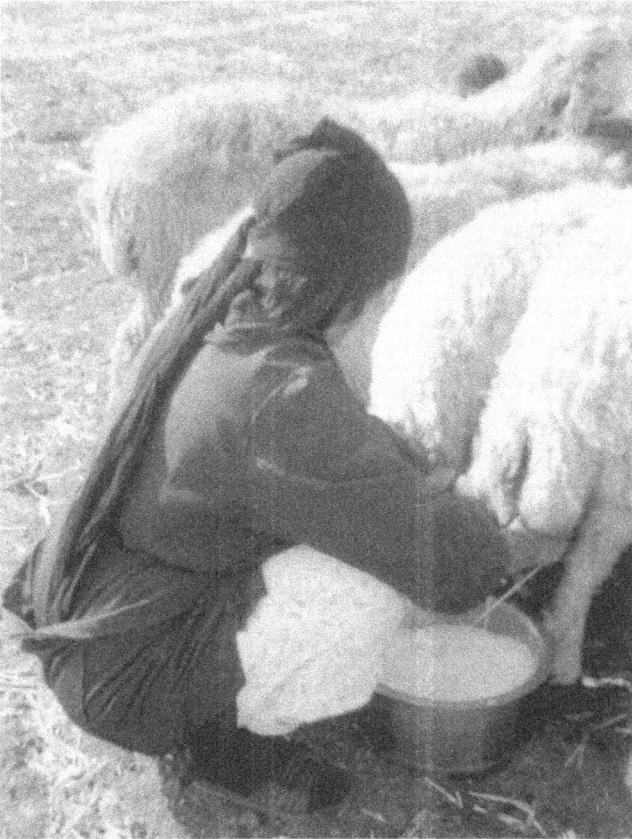

Figures 3.4 a. and b. Bedouin woman roping and milking sheep as her daughter watches.

nese pounds. Bedouin are thus tied to the larger capitalist system, because the price of milk, crop residues, and feedstuffs is determined by regional and international markets. In the spring, pastoralists shear the sheep and sell the wool to regional merchants and mattress-making factories.

Although Bedouin pastoralists have control of the means of production in terms of livestock, grazing land is usually secured through contracts with peasant landowners. Bedouin pastoralists are semisedentary, and access to grazing lands in the summer (June–September) and spring (March–May) is largely secured by paid contracts (oral, not written) with peasant landowners. That is, Bedouin livestock owners in the summertime pay per dunum to graze their flocks on the stubble left after crops are harvested—the price of harvest yields is determined by harvest crop. Because some of the land on mountain slopes is not individually owned but public or abandoned land, every now and then, pastoralists can graze their flocks in the spring at no cost. In the winter and, periodically, in the spring, Bedouin rely on purchased feedstuffs. Some herd owners also purchase vitamins in the winter. To protect their flocks from the cold and rainy winter season, Bedouin pastoralists place their herds in cement enclosures or small makeshift barns. Pastoral households in 2000 moved about twice per year on average—once in the summer and once in the spring—which requires combined dwellings (i.e., tent and permanent house). Households migrate as a unit, or else husband and wife migrate together and leave some children to stay behind under the protection of extended family members or older siblings. Spouses are rarely separated for long periods of time.

The current Bedouin economic structure reflects political-economic developments that began in the mid-twentieth century (see chapter 2). Over the last five decades, Bedouins have become increasingly sedentary and rely less on economic pastoralism and more on farming and wage labor for their livelihoods. The skewed distribution of Bedouin livestock (sheep/goats and cows) holdings and land holdings points to economic differentiation within Bedouin communities (see tables 3.1–3.4). Table 3.5 shows that access to the means of production varies by occupational group. Pastoral households are in the most favorable situation of all the economic groups. It is not too surprising that 95.3 percent of Bedouin households classified as pastoralists (whose dominant economic mode of production since marriage is pastoralism) own sheep and goats. Approximately 71.9 percent of pastoralists own trucks. Pastoral households are also in the most favorable situation of all the economic groups in terms of ownership of land (although holdings are minuscule). Sharecroppers/tenant farmers and other/miscellaneous occupations are in the middle range of productive wealth ownership,

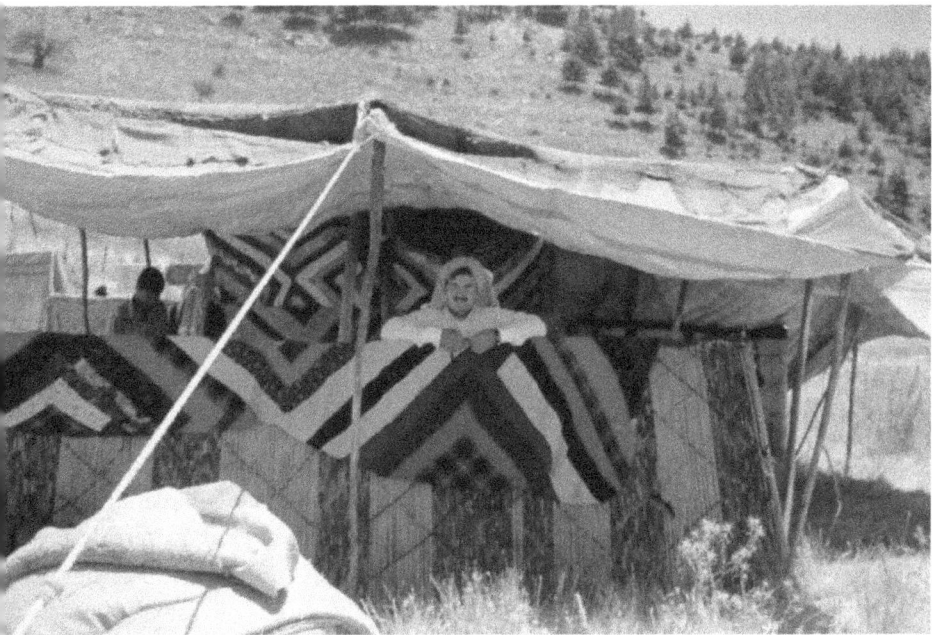

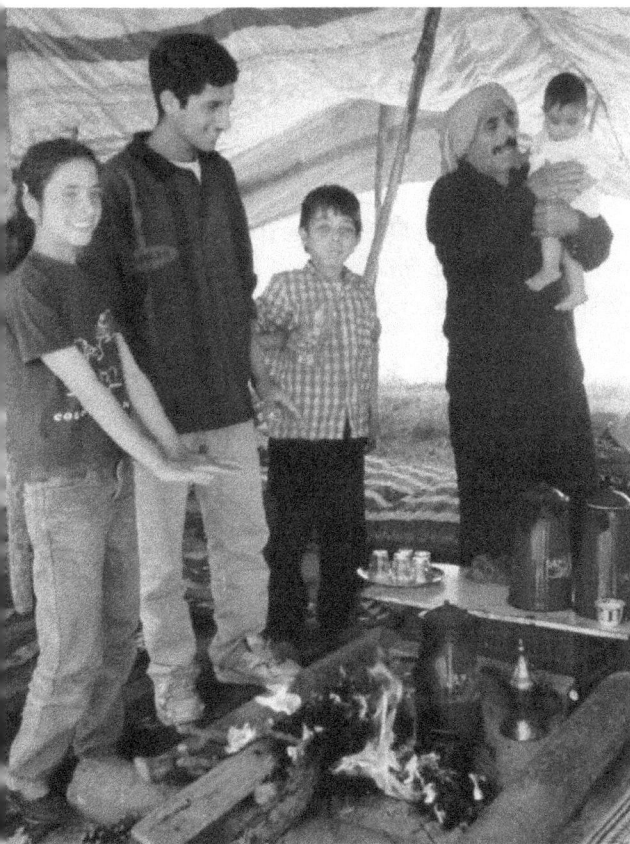

Figures 3.5 a. and b. Bedouin pastoral household in their spring tent.

Table 3.5. Household ownership status of the means of production by occupation, 2000–2001

| | (% Yes) Means of Production | | | | | | |
Occupation	Land	Sheep/Goats	Cows	Trucks	Cars	Tractors	Generators
Pastoralists	46.9	95.3	6.3	71.9	9.4	1.6	3.1
Sharecroppers/ Tenant Farmers	25.0	21.0	13.0	63.0	6.0	12.0	3.0
Wage Laborers	15.4	29.2	7.7	18.5	10.8	1.5	0.0
Other	36.4	27.3	36.4	72.7	18.2	0.0	0.0

Note: N = 240 households.

although those involved in other/miscellaneous work are slightly better off. Sharecroppers have the highest rate of tractor ownership at 12 percent. Wage laborers are in the least favorable position in terms of overall ownership of the means of production. However, when it comes to ownership of herd animals, roughly 29.2 percent of wage-laborer households own at least some sheep/goats. Ownership of machinery, such as tractors and generators, is extremely rare.

These data should be considered in conjunction with information presented earlier in this chapter on Bedouin ownership of the means of production. The majority of Bedouin households do not own land, sheep/goats, or cows. What is more, Bedouin livestock holdings among pastoralists are often insufficient to support a family. Bedouin estimate that a herd of at least one hundred fifty is needed to support a family of five or six, hence less than half of those who own livestock (43.5 percent) have a herd adequate to support a family (see table 3.3). For this reason, most Bedouin pastoralists rely on multiple forms of economic activity, such as occasional sharecropping or tenancy and wage labor, for survival. Both pastoralist and sharecropping families depend on the income derived from the wage labor of adolescent youth and girls in particular. Hence, the proletarianization of child labor is an important feature of the Bedouin social economy.

Bedouin Demographic Structure

One of the main questions for anthropological demographers and other social theorists interested in transnational and historical processes of class formation is whether or not distinct forms of production—pastoralism, sharecropping, and wage labor, in the Bedouin case—have given rise to class tensions and class-specific demographic regimes.[27] Table 3.6 shows

Table 3.6. Mean number of live births and survivors by occupation among 102 postreproductive Bedouin women

Occupation	No.	Mean Live Births	Mean Survivors
Pastoralism	36	9.5 ± 3.5	8.5 ± 3.1
Wage Labor	25	9.4 ± 2.3	8.6 ± 2.2
Sharecropping/Tenant	37	8.5 ± 2.6	7.9 ± 2.4
Other	4	8.8 ± 1.0	8.5 ± 0.6
Total	102	9.1 ± 2.9	8.3 ± 2.6

the number of live births and survivors for 102 postreproductive Bedouin women in different occupational groups. These women were either interviewed in 2000–2001 or 2007, but all were postreproductive or near postreproductive by the year 2000. Pastoralists and wage laborers have slightly higher fertility than sharecroppers, but the differences are minor. Likewise, there is little demographic variation in the number of survivors across occupational groups. Of the three main occupational groups, sharecroppers have the highest survivorship (and lowest average number of child deaths) and pastoralists have the lowest survivorship (and highest average number of child deaths), although the disparities are small and not statistically significant. Similar results were obtained when examining mortality outcomes of 1,399 births (1,110 births after exclusions) to 240 Bedouin women (aged fifteen to fifty-four years) interviewed in 2000–2001. Mortality rates were examined for both infants (less than twelve months old) and children (twelve to fifty-nine months old) and reveal an absence of significant occupational and wealth differentials in infant and child mortality within Bekaa Bedouin communities. An unexpected finding to emerge from these analyses is that the small observed differences in early child mortality between the economic groups are not even in the predicted direction. Greater wealth is associated with higher, not lower, mortality, although the association became insignificant when appropriate statistical controls were included.[28] A likely explanation for this pattern is that wealthier families who possess a greater number of domestic animals may face a heightened risk of child death as a result of infection from specifically animal pathogens and the increased prevalence of zoonotic parasites.

The absence of socioeconomic differentials is particularly important given evidence of class tensions and class-specific demographic differentials between landowning peasants and land-poor Bedouin in the Bekaa Valley, with Bedouin having higher fertility and mortality. There are several plausible explanations as to why economic differences have not translated into mortality differences within Bedouin communities. First, Bedouins of varying economic means appear to have benefited from the availability of clean (uncontaminated) and reliable sources of water in the Bekaa Valley, Lebanon. Second, the Bedouin have at least some access (no matter how limited) to the extensive network of clinics and primary health centers in Lebanon. Finally, as discussed above, there are sociocultural practices that serve to prevent economic exploitation and even out existing economic disparities between social strata. Generous and extensive Bedouin food-sharing has important implications for child health (see below). Children enjoy meals with extended family members in their village, particularly their father's brother's families, on a weekly, if not daily, basis.

Economic inequality by itself does not constitute class division. Economic inequalities are not necessarily "permanent," as one's status and wealth can fluctuate considerably through time (see chapter 8). Sociocultural forms of economic redistribution can also even out economic disparities. A major criterion for the designation of class relations is that the former entails exploitative social relationships where use of a surplus product by a group that has not contributed the corresponding surplus of labor reproduces the conditions of a new extortion of surplus labor from the producers.[29] In the Bekaa, one group (peasants) has control of the means of production utilized by the other group (Bedouin), giving rise to a relationship of inequality and class stratification. The ownership of land, which is the basis of class exploitation, is in the hands of peasant proprietors, limiting opportunities for hierarchy at the local level. In other words, the Bedouin, for the most part, do not own the means of production for entering into exploitative economic relationships. Without land, it is not possible to "hire in" agricultural wage laborers or arrange for sharecroppers to perform labor in exchange for a portion of the crop. Similarly, Bedouin pastoralists rely on grazing land rented from peasant landowners and purchased feed produced in industrial factories to sustain their herds. In terms of labor, pastoralists predominantly rely on family labor for herding; that is, they do not "hire in" the labor of other Lebanese Bedouin. On the flip side, Lebanese Bedouin generally do not "hire out," or sell their labor as a commodity, to other Bedouin (it is seen as dishonorable), which has thus far prevented exploitative relations from emerging within Lebanese Bedouin communities.

It is possible that what we might be witnessing here are the very beginnings of class formation within Bekaa Bedouin communities. As economic disparities become more entrenched, they may give rise to future class and health disparities at the local level. Lebanese Bedouin pastoralists could begin hiring Lebanese Bedouin shepherds to tend to their animals, paving the way toward more exploitative relations in the future. However, there is also another possibility, namely that Bedouin who enjoy greater ownership of the means of production may find themselves increasingly joining the ranks of poorer families. Many wage laborers in 2000 worked as pastoralists just a decade ago. They sold their flocks to meet the costs of home construction and sedentary life. Bad years owing to difficult political-economic circumstances may force families in the future to sell their livestock holdings. Families could also incur substantial livestock losses, as they did in the recent 2006 summer war, making it difficult to maintain the minimum number of livestock needed to pursue a viable economic existence as pastoralists. Institutionalized discrimination of Bedouin only adds to the precariousness of their economic situation.

Either way, at this particular point in time, it is noteworthy that economic distinctions within Bedouin communities have not translated into either fertility or early-child-mortality differentials, which suggest a reproductive experience distinct from that of women in more stratified peasant and pastoral societies (see chapters 7 and 8). It is frequently assumed that in small-scale geographically peripheral communities with similar ethnic composition and strong kinship bonds, like those of the Bedouin, socioeconomic differentials in health will be minimal and outweighed by biogenetic factors. The relative importance of biogenetic factors in shaping health outcomes varies according to social and ecological circumstances. Public-health researchers observe that biogenetic factors are generally less important in contexts where environmental conditions known to negatively impact health are widespread. For example in global South countries with pervasive malnutrition and infectious diseases linked to suboptimal child growth, the heritability of height is lower. Likewise, biogenetic factors are likely to be more important in contexts where environmental conditions (e.g., malnutrition and infectious disease) known to affect health are least present. A Finnish study examining the heritability of height across four birth cohorts found that as living conditions in Finland improved, the heritability of height increased.[30] As certain groups or communities (well-off middle-class groups in global North and South countries) undergo the epidemiological transition and see a reduction in socioeconomic disparities in health, public-health researchers predict that the role of biological and genetic factors in determining morbidity and mortality will become increasingly important.[31]

The sociodemographic markings of class are absent within Bedouin communities, which leads us to expect a more prominent role for biogenetic influences on health. In terms of early child health, I was able to identify three salient determinants of early mortality: birth interval, birth order, and consanguinity. The most important factor affecting Bedouin infant and child mortality is birth interval, which is largely determined by breastfeeding duration. A short preceding birth interval is associated with increased infant- and child-mortality risk among the Bedouin. Data collected on the outcome of 1,399 births (1,110 births after exclusions) to 240 Bedouin women in 2000–2001 shows that the mean birth interval is 25.1 months, and for every one-month increase in preceding birth interval, the adjusted odds of child death decreases by a factor of 0.963, or 3.7 percent.[32] The detrimental impact of short preceding birth intervals on infant and child mortality is well established in the demographic literature.[33] While short birth spacing was found to be significantly associated with an increased risk of mortality in both infancy (less than twelve months old) and childhood (twelve to fifty-nine completed months), birth order and consanguineous marriage were found to increase the risk of mortality only during infancy.[34]

Later-born Bedouin children are at a higher mortality risk than earlier-born children.[35] There are several possible explanations for this pattern. First, children born into large families may have less access to parental time and care, which may affect the level of attention given to the health and safety of children during the first year of life. The problem with this explanation is that it undermines the caretaking contributions of older children as well as extended family members. Another more plausible possibility is that children born into an already large family in a house filled with siblings face a greater risk of exposure to infectious disease, especially given that they have not yet fully acquired their own immunity. The third explanation centers on maternal, or biological, depletion as women age and experience successive pregnancies. However, in the Bedouin case, maternal age was not found to be a significant predictor of either infant or child mortality.

Consanguineous marriage (defined for purposes of the analysis as marriage between first cousins) was also found to have a significant negative impact on Bedouin infant mortality. The deleterious impact of consanguinity is largely due to homozygosity for deleterious recessive alleles. If two people who possess the same harmful recessive gene mate, then one out of every four children will get two copies of the bad gene (one from the father and one from the mother) and develop the genetic disorder. Numerous harmful recessive disorders have been documented, including mental retardation, birth defects, and nervous-system disorders. Many of these disorders are believed to be fatal early in life. Among the Bekaa Bedouin, infants born to first cousins have more than double (2.2) the odds of dying than infants born to nonfirst-cousin couples.[36] The health risks of close-kin marriage in Bedouin society must be kept in perspective. The National Society of Genetic Counselors has tried to put that risk in context for cousin couples. Children of nonrelated couples have a 2–3 percent risk of birth defects as opposed to first cousins, who have a 4–6 percent risk. First cousins thus have over a 94 percent chance of having healthy children. In the general population, the risk that a child will be born with a serious problem like spina bifida or cystic fibrosis is 3–4 percent; to that background risk, first cousins must add another 1.7 to 2.8 percentage points.[37] This is about the same risk that a pregnant woman over the age of 40 faces in having a baby with birth defects. The health risks of consanguinity must also be considered in conjunction with the social, political, psychological, and emotional benefits to marrying kin (see chapter 5 for a better understanding of marriage between relatives).

When considering the impact of consanguineous marriage or birth spacing, it is important to recognize that these are sociocultural practices with important underlying biological effects. A scalar or hierarchical approach recognizes that broader levels provide context and help explain why a pattern exists, whereas finer levels provide mechanistic or how explanations. Recessive-gene expression in close consanguineous progeny is the biological mechanism by which consanguineous marriage can elevate early mortality. Mechanisms need not be entirely biological. For example, if close-kin couples were found to have less access to social and economic resources that provide a health advantage, then it would be necessary to include socioeconomic mechanisms in proximate explanations of mortality. It is possible to make analytical distinctions between nature and society while acknowledging that both are interdependent and dynamically exist in reciprocal relation to one another.

As demographers and health researchers with a biocultural bent, we must be careful not to be blindsided by biogenetic factors in our efforts to understand the determinants of child health. Limits to knowledge due to data limitations also need to be taken into account. This is especially true for marginalized and effectively stateless groups like the Bedouin who are largely excluded from vital registration systems. Autopsy or cause-of-death statistics from reliable health facilities are regarded as the most reliable sources of data for ascertaining cause of death (although they are not without problems). The current study relies on parental reports and demographic statistics derived from Bedouin reproductive histories as its main source of data on early child mortality. If we examine epidemiological data from Lebanon in 2007 (the time of my second field visit), the data reveal that most reported cases of death for children under five, at the national level, were due to measles—an infectious disease, followed by typhoid fever and dysentery, which are food- and water-borne diseases.[38] Information on reported deaths by region (the data for regions is not broken down by age) indicates that most deaths in the Bekaa were due to food- and water-borne illnesses, with typhoid fever being the most common, and viral hepatitis A and brucellosis representing the second- and third-most common causes of death, respectively.[39] Cause-of-death information obtained from Bedouin reproductive histories were sometimes difficult to interpret, as many parents stated unknown or supernatural causes of child death. There were, however, several reported child deaths due to accidents, which included children falling down wells, burning alive as a result of tents catching on fire, electrocution, run-over accidents caused by farm tractors, and death due to war-related injuries. Accidents do not appear to have abated with the epidemiological transition, which means that we should take pause before declaring the waning impact of sociotechnological factors on health in societies where economic disparities in health are minimal. Given that the demographic markings of class are absent and the economic markings of class are present, albeit somewhat low at the local level, what can we conclude about social equality and social-status distinctions within Bedouin communities?

Tribe and Class

I opened the chapter with a discussion of the class tensions between Bedouin and peasants and cultural differences between the groups. It is impossible to overlook Bedouin-peasant class tensions in the Bekaa, as they are an ever-present reality. It surprised me that in conversations about peasants, Bedouins downplayed or minimized class cleavages. More often than not, individuals avoided the subject, changed the subject and took the exact opposite view, focusing instead on their religious and cultural commonalities with peasant groups. As I think back on these dialogues, it is possible to see them as common strategies, even cultural forms of avoidance or "dialogic repression,"[40] that individuals and groups employ to reduce personal/political anxiety and pain resulting from inhospitable conditions of their cultural-historical environment. We know that it was a widespread social practice among Jews in Europe to avoid discussing anti-Semitism and oppression within their society. As a socially marginalized minority within the Bekaa, Bedouins must continually confront oppression and develop strategies both individually and socially for coping with those interpersonal challenges associated with prejudice in peasant society.

With that said, classlike tensions within Bedouin communities of the Bekaa Valley are conspicuous for their absence. In spite of my probing during work-history interviews, Bedouin women and men showed little interest in discussing classlike tensions within Bedouin communities. I was not easily deterred. I pressed on with my questions for months. My interlocutors tried their best to accommodate my interests, even encouraging me by saying, "Yes, write that down; there are differences in wealth. Good." Conversations about internal social differences always shifted from class to tribe. Social class was not a topic avoided by Bedouin, but one that held little or no interest. Ethnographic accounts of social structure among Bedouin peoples and other segmentary groups in the Middle East and North Africa have long been described with egalitarian phrases like "balanced rivalry,"[41] "ordered anarchy,"[42] and "complementary opposition"[43] (see chapter 8 for a comparative discussion of social equalities and inequalities in nomadic societies).

Because I began interviews for my fieldwork in the North Bekaa and gradually made my way south, it took several weeks to meet families from different tribes. The most visible marker of tribal affiliation is women's dress. Different tribes have different styles of veiling. Initially, I thought that rank or hierarchy were clearly defined, based on cultural forms of dress among women and the fact that my interlocutors would confidently assert, "Our 'ashīra (tribe/clan) is the best 'ashīra. We are honest; we are generous and have the best reputation." It was only after a month or so that I began to realize that members of different tribes made virtually identical pronouncements about their own tribe's social standing and honor. Bedouin women and men enjoyed questioning me as to which tribe I liked the best. In typical fashion, we would be drinking tea and socializing after an interview, and I would be asked, "In learning about Bedouin life, you have traveled and seen all the tribes in the Bekaa. Tell us, which tribe do you like the best?" This question was always asked with a sense of curiosity and amusement. There is no indigenous attempt or interest in ranking tribes. Further, while individuals recognize wealthier families and tribes (e.g., those who possess sizable livestock holdings), economic advantage has not led to socially recognized status hierarchies or hierarchical differences in possession of honor. Individuals from different tribes did not put down or denigrate other tribes or describe them as socially inferior, but rather were more concerned with asserting their own tribe's honor and virtuousness. Honor is horizontally diffused, not vertically concentrated, in Bedouin communities. Even tribal shaykhs or chiefs are not recognized as being of superior social rank. Bedouin men and women criticize shaykhs whose personal skills and character they judge to be deficient (referring to them as liars) and praise others for their more adept arbitration skills. The sociopolitical role of shaykhs is that of mediators with potential skills to be utilized by *all* members for solving disputes and social problems.

In addition to honor, the central tribal values emphasized by Bedouin in speech and practice are generosity and hospitality. Numerous practices and expressions demonstrate Bedouin attention to these values. It is considered important to "*raḥḥab bī l-dayf*" (welcome the guest hospitably), display *shahama* (magnanimity/chivalry/generosity), and treat neighbors in accordance with these values so that there is no *ḥiqd* (spite/rancor/grudge/malice) between them. Food-sharing is one of the most visible manifestations of Bedouin generosity. Bedouins believe that it is morally wrong to deny children and pregnant women food. The sharing of food extends to nursing of infants. Caring for and nursing other people's children are reciprocal acts of kindness extended to both kin and nonkin. One of my informants described the difficulties of being reared without a biological mother (she died an hour after he was born), but details the efforts of his kinship circle and community to nurse him:

> My father's sister's daughter is about two months older than I am. We were breastfed together. I was nursed by my father's sister. But before I got to my father's sister [let me go back to the beginning] . . . A human being should be clear in explaining everything. When it comes to my wife, my children, and my friends, they tell me that my *'āṣabiyya* (nerves/temperament/tribal spirit) is *shadīd* (strong/powerful/vigorous) and stubborn. When I was first born, I was nursed by a Gypsy woman. That is one. When I was first born after my mother died, I was nursed by a Gypsy and she filled my stomach. They put me there. I got hungry. [After that] I was nursed by a black woman. Again I got hungry. [Next] I was nursed by a Bedouin woman. Then they delivered me to my father's sister. My father's sister . . . her husband is Kurdish. Her milk is the milk of the Kurds. The milk is coarse. Yes, my father's sister raised me in this life. For this reason, my *akhlāq* (character/moral constitution) is difficult, *sharis* (quarrelsome/pugnacious/petulant) and stubborn. [laughs] Leave it to Allāh! My father's sister nursed me for one year and a half.

Cross-nursing by relatives and neighbors is often reported in Bedouin reproductive histories. Breast milk is an important mediator of character and kinship. The health benefits of breastfeeding discussed previously are well known. Cross-nursing is a customary practice that improves a child's life chances by extending the benefits of breastfeeding to those children whose mothers died during childbirth or were otherwise unable to nurse them (due to an inability to produce sufficient breast milk, for example).

The strong presence of communal sharing and generosity do not imply that social tensions or divisions between kin or tribal members are absent. Maintaining good kinship relations through hospitality, visiting, and sharing requires sufficient expenditure of time, energy, and resources. Tensions are even visible at the most basic levels of kinship. Sometimes these tensions erupt into violence, as when a brother killed his male sibling and that sibling's eldest son during a dispute over grazing almost a decade prior to my first visit to the Bekaa in 2000. Of particular relevance to this confrontation is the fact that the murdered brother was married to a woman from a different tribe (see chapter 5 for a discussion of kinship ties). While fighting or confrontation between brothers and other close relatives is not uncommon—a matter well understood by the classic tragedians—fighting only rarely leads to killing. This particular double homicide is one of the few[44] preserved in the living memories of Bedouin in the Bekaa. The brother who committed the murders was strongly censured by his living brothers, other paternal kin, and tribal community. The dispute was resolved through mediation by a well-respected tribal shaykh from Syria. The brother who committed the murders was not allowed to speak to the victim's wife or children. The shaykh, in conjunction with the broader tribal community, ordered that the offender make an enormous "satisfaction payment" to the widow and her children (in the amount of approximately 15 million Lebanese pounds) in order to compensate them for their loss and to prevent further violence in the community. The requirement that injured parties be compensated helps protect the weak and places limits on individuals or groups who are more powerful, physically stronger, aggressive, or simply reckless. Tribes have shared guidelines for proper human conduct designed to prevent certain individuals from dominating others.

Conclusion

At this early stage of peasantization, there is little evidence of either classlike tensions or occupation-specific demographic differentials within Bedouin communities. Class tensions, class exploitation, and class-specific demographic differentials are apparent at different scales, most notably between Bedouins and peasants.[45] Demographic and economic inequities between Bedouin and peasant groups are easily discernable, with the former having higher birth and death rates as well as less landed wealth. The classist dis-respect directed towards Bedouins, at least by rural peasants in the Bekaa, is not expressed in the European Malthusian language of sexual laxity, hy-perfecundity, and poverty. Bedouin poverty is not contemptuous in and of itself. Poverty is at best only indirectly invoked, in discourses on bodily cleanliness—which have strong religious and racial connotations. Likewise, the Bedouin are not directly scorned by peasants for their high fertility, but admonished for not following normative child-rearing practices with regard to education—a reproach that has class connotations.

Within their own Bedouin communities, exploitative classlike conflicts are less apparent. Even though economic disparities between Bedouin pas-toralists, sharecroppers, and wage laborers are visible, demographic dispari-ties in fertility and mortality between the occupational groups are not. The Bedouin have maintained egalitarianism through sociocultural practices that emphasize generosity, cooperation, and sharing. Whether it be cultural codes of work and honor that prevent the sale of Bedouin labor to other Bedouin, traditions of hospitality, food-sharing, or other forms of economic assistance, adherence to these cultural beliefs in practice has helped deter the spread of potentially exploitative social relations. Moreover, contrary to expectations that health worsens as one's economic standing declines, neither wealth (operationalized in terms of ownership of the means of pro-duction) nor occupational status has a measurable effect on child health within Bedouin communities. The Bedouin young who face a heightened risk of death are the infants and children born after short birth intervals, the infants born to consanguineous parents, and the children born later in the birth order. To speak of "stratified reproduction" can be misleading, as it implies that individuals are already *universally* constituted as a group with fixed class, gender, and racial identities. Class inequality is not a fixed or in-evitable feature of human societies. Class differences are uneven in time and place. The next chapter pays closer attention to demographic distinctions of gender, exposing the colonial myths underlying interpretations of women's high fertility.

4

Gender Myths and Demographic Realities

Homogenous narratives of Arab women's and other Third World women's patriarchal oppression are part of a historically long and geographically wide colonial legacy. Western colonialism and feminism converge in their concerns over Third World women's fertility being too high. The reproduction of Arab-Muslim bodies in particular constitutes a demographic threat to colonial and imperial agendas.[1] High fertility is seen by Western feminists through a similar negative prism of Third World women's subjugation at the hands of Third World men. By depicting Arab fertility as dangerously high and contiguously linked to militant religious fundamentalism and male-on-female domination, popular and academic narratives provide cover for colonialism.[2] Anthropological demographers are beginning to challenge colonial myths of gender, reproduction, and family life on empirical and interpretive grounds.[3] In Bedouin communities of the Bekaa Valley where fertility is high, I assess how women and men articulate the value of children while establishing the empirical parameters of variation in women's completed fertility. By attending to gender disparities in health as well as the cultural importance of large families among older cohorts of Bedouin women, we are in a better position to address (classist, racist, and sexist) misconceptions about high fertility embedded in Western feminist accounts. I begin by briefly reviewing some of the colonial myths of gender that have influenced our perceptions of Third World women's reproduction.

Colonial Myths of Gender and Fertility

In order to understand why high fertility is persistently articulated by Western feminists through the idiom of oppression, we must trace the coalescence of feminism and colonialism. Leila Ahmed historically traces this coming together of feminism and colonialism in Western discourse on Islam and finds that colonial narratives began to place women's "oppression" at the center of their prose in the late nineteenth century.[4] It was at this time that colonial Britain developed its eugenicist and social Darwinian theories of race and evolutionary progress with middle-class Victorian England serving as the pinnacle of civilization. A body of knowledge and scholarship was produced, especially the emergent study of anthropology, to legitimize European superiority and its colonial subjugation of "inferior" non-European peoples. While the Victorian male elite rejected the application of feminist ideas such as patriarchy and oppression to interpret their own behavior, they were more than eager to use pseudofeminist language as a weapon against other peoples, particularly nonwhite men. Ahmed explains:

> It was here and in the combining of the languages of colonialism and feminism that the fusion between the issues of women and culture was created. More exactly, what was created was the fusion between the issues of women, their oppression, and the cultures of Other men. The idea that Other men, men in colonized societies or societies beyond the borders of the civilized West, oppressed women was to be used, in the rhetoric of colonialism, to render morally justifiable its project of undermining or eradicating the cultures of colonized peoples.[5]

Ahmed calls this colonial cooption of feminist language "colonial feminism." Feminist rhetoric is used as an instrument of colonial power and domination. Demonization and dehumanization of Arab men provides justification for white colonial conquest.

In the Americas, Andrea Smith shows how Euramerican colonists relied on similar tropes to subjugate indigenous nations. Indian men were depicted as murderous savages abducting white women and dominating Indian women, when in reality it was white men who were perpetrating Indian genocide and sexual violence against Indian women. The artifice of colonial history was used to conceal white rape of Native women and construct Indian men as the oppressors. Smith writes:

> Ironically, while enslaving women's bodies, colonizers argued that they were actually somehow freeing Native women from the "oppression" they supposedly faced in Native nations. Thomas Jefferson argued that Native women "are submitted to unjust drudgery. This I believe is the case with every barbarous people. It is civilization alone which replaces women in the enjoyment of their equality."[6]

The Euramerican conception of freedom requires that Native women be colonized, and thereby rendered unfree, in order to be made "free." It is clear that freedom has a twisted colonial connotation. Freedom is united with its opposite: domination. Native women must be "liberated" from Native men, much like Arab women need to be "liberated" from Arab men,[7] so that they are "free" to be controlled by white colonial society. Ahmed observes that inferiority was imposed differently on colonized societies. Hence, Western feminism as the handmaiden of colonialism was "tailored to fit the particular culture that was the immediate target of domination—India, the Islamic world, sub-Saharan Africa."[8] What we see is the same imperial principle of divide and conquer constituted in diverse ways and used to pit women against men (in addition to tribe against tribe; race against race; and religion against religion).

With respect to women's reproduction, both Western imperialism and Western feminism espouse negative views of high fertility. On the one hand, high fertility is linked to fears of overpopulation, which is deeply inculcated in the ongoing history of imperialism and decolonization. European fertility had already begun to decline in the final decades of the nineteenth century, but fertility in Arab countries, and the Third World in general, remained high until the 1960s.[9] Imperial authorities in the 1930s and 1940s became aware that population was growing in their overseas colonies in North Africa, India, Indochina, Korea, and the West and East Indies. Colonial officials partly blamed the fall of empire on population growth. In the era of decolonization, many "feared a further redistribution of wealth and power between rich and poor, in which metropoles would lose access to oil and other natural resources, or even suffer reverse 'colonization' by migrants from former possessions now grown overpopulated."[10] Western feminism also problematizes high fertility. One of the long-standing colonial feminist myths about women's fertility that is almost never questioned even by progressive Western feminists otherwise critical of overpopulation rhetoric is the assumption that high fertility—when and where it does occur—is emblematic of the patriarchal subordination of women.

A progressive feminist classic on the global politics of reproduction describes high Third World fertility as follows: "In many Third World countries the economic subordination of women is directly linked to high birth rates, since it both increases their need for children and impedes their ability to practice birth control."[11] The subordination of women and their lack of freedom are believed to stem directly from bearing and raising children. From this Western feminist standpoint, children stand in the way of women's economic independence and obstruct them from using birth control. Women's interests are pitted against those of their children. Such an ideology encourages the separation of women from their families and communities. Economic interdependency is replaced by the notion of dependency, which has negative connotations of weakness and passivity. While Western feminists generally support women's control over their own reproduction, it remains difficult for most to accept that Third World women who have large families are not invariably dominated by their husbands or victims of a patriarchal society. In keeping with the unshakable assumption of Third World women's victimization, we are further told that "a child pleases a woman's husband and her in-laws, the people who control her life."[12] The underlying premise is that Third World women find little pleasure and meaning in children. Women are believed to be controlled by their families, especially their husbands. Because Third World women's reproductive lives are believed to be dictated by the fear of "widowhood, divorce, or abandonment," it is asserted that "many women need children" for economic and old-age support.[13] Third World women's economic and emotional reliance on their families is viewed as one-way and nonreciprocal. The Third World family is metaphorized and metamorphosed into a woman's prison.

The secular progressive goal advanced by white middle-class feminists is based on a specific notion of individual liberty or autonomy.[14] Western society's dependence on government services and entitlement programs is not questioned or problematized. For Western feminists, it is the extended family and children that supposedly keep Third World women down. Western women are not depicted as subordinate, dependent, or weak. Submission to and dependence on the nation-state is considered normative and not seen as an obstruction to women's freedom or independence. In contrast, Third World women's reliance on the family and community is marshaled as evidence of their subordinate status. These Western representations of Third World women are ubiquitous to the point of being hegemonic.

Colonial feminist constructions of individual liberty are based on racial, class, *and* gender polarity. Gender polarity refers to the idealization of "masculine" individuality and derogation of "feminine" dependency. Jessica Benjamin has argued that "individuation based on denying the need for others is hardly liberation," but serves to reinforce gender splitting and domination.[15] Chandra Mohanty has challenged constructions of Third World women as devoid of agency and victims of "tradition." Third World women are discursively constructed as passive and agentless victims in reference to "free" Western women who are believed to be in control over their lives. Mohanty refers to this hegemonic codification of Third World women in scholarship as "discursive" colonization.[16] More recently, Sarah Hoagland has developed the concept of "heterosexualism" to explain constructed gender binaries and the various ways women are expected to subordinate themselves to men.[17] The constructed categories of "men" and "women" help re-create patriarchy and white supremacy. White men and white women are "the standard of men and women by which everyone else is measured and falls short in one way or another (too fat, not white [enough], not feminine enough, not masculine enough, too old, not bearing children, and so on)."[18] Through the writings of critical feminist theorists, we are reminded that nonwhite women have different gender experiences, although their experiences exist in historical dialogue with each other and with those of white women. Chapter 3 shows that Arab women's fertility in Lebanon varies even within the same rural setting. In the Bekaa Valley, the reproductive experiences of Bedouin Arab women differ from those of non-Bedouin Arab women. The differences relate to divergent classlike experiences and histories, particularly with respect to seminomadic pastoralism.

Perspectives that undermine women's agency fail to recognize that social structures are produced and reproduced by individuals and groups of individuals, or, conversely, that in and through their actions, women draw upon social structures and reconstitute them in the process. Structure and agency intersect through praxis, and should be studied empirically. In the next section, I take up questions pertaining to gender relations and gender-specific demographic disparities. I then turn to Bedouin discursive accounts of childbearing in order to provide greater insight into actors' inclinations and the conditions of action that produce large, medium, small, and childless families.

Gender Relations and Demographic Disparities

The most personally unsettling aspect of being in the field that took the most time to adjust to was gender relations, but not for the reasons commonly assumed. I remember being uncomfortable and disoriented for the first several months. I had come face to face with proud, fearless, and strong women and did not know what to make of gender realities that conflicted with my expectations. I watched in disbelief as women aggressively silenced their husbands or dismissed their opinions and asserted their own voices. I listened as women teased their husbands (in front of kin and neighbors) with highly inflammatory remarks and watched everyone laugh it off with ease. Indeed, men did not get upset and no fighting ensued over women's boldness. It is naïve to assume that for a Western-educated Arab woman growing up in the United States and confronting a gender egalitarian Bedouin social order that my initial reaction would be one of liberation or joy. The first several nights that I spent with a Bedouin family, I had difficulty sleeping. I stayed up most of the night listening, trying to determine if the husband was going to get into an argument with his wife. As soon as everyone was up in the morning, I would study the faces and demeanor of my hosts, looking for signs of gender trouble. I remember thinking that I was missing something and that sooner or later the bubble would burst and I would be confronted with the more sinister but "real" face of male patriarchy.

That women subordinate themselves to men is not a taken-for-granted assumption or expectation in Bedouin society. Bedouin femininity is not synonymous with dependency, subservience, and compliance. Men recognize that their wives are not extensions of themselves and have independent and sometimes conflicting interests. Women are relaxed in the company of their husbands. The fact that a close familiarity marks spousal relationships is not too surprising, considering the frequency of Bedouin marriages between relatives (see chapter 5). Bedouin men publicly acknowledge the value of their wives in terms of the hard work they perform and the companionship they provide. Bedouin husbands feel no shame or discomfort in voicing or showing their appreciation and affection for their wives. Physical displays of intimacy in public are not common, but there are other ways of physically communicating love and affection. When I gave a Bedouin couple the photos I had taken of them and their family, the husband picked up the two photos of his wife, placing one in each hand, and took turns pressing each photo to his lips. It is important not to ignore the role of age in determining women's status vis-à-vis men. As women age and become senior members of their community, they are socially recognized for their greater wisdom and counsel. However, it was also clear that women at younger ages do not lack social confidence. Women begin helping out their families as laborers in their early teens. Their demeanor even at an earlier age is marked by bold maturity and confidence. They participate in social conversations comfortably. And while they heed their mothers and fathers on many matters, they are not afraid to challenge parental authority.

Some discernable changes in gender relations appear to have accompanied peasantization. The replacement of camels with pickup trucks has altered the cultural structuring of gender relations. Bedouin women traditionally decorated camels and rode on them. Although women ride in pickup trucks and other vehicles today, they do not drive them. Trucks are socially and symbolically tied to men and exclude women from an important mode of transportation used to support the household economy. Trucks create new gender divisions and separation of spheres within the social order, as Bedouin men are afforded greater mobility and access to peasant life in a way that women are not. Changes in religious organization and practice have also accompanied the transition to settled life. Bedouin nomadism prevented regular attendance at mosque, especially during Friday prayers when mosques are filled with worshippers. Most mosques in the Bekaa accommodate women who can pray in a separate partitioned area. For the most part, however, Bedouin women pray at home. They do not attend mosque as frequently as men, which limits their public participation in an important religious activity.

In looking for other visible manifestations of gender inequities in daily life, I could not help but notice the muted form of gender segregation in Bedouin households. Bedouin men and women usually sit together on futonlike mattresses placed on the floor. It is customary to sit close together with arms propped up on a shared pillow so that one cannot help but rub elbows with the person seated next to him or her. Family members often eat together, and husbands and wives as well as male and female siblings frequently share the same plate or bowl. Women's veiling is sometimes taken as evidence of greater female seclusion and modesty, but men too are veiled in Bedouin society. Cultural values of modesty and honor require covering most parts of the body, except for the hands and face. The gender-related distinctions that I observed were mostly confined to the households of prominent shaykhs. Women married to shaykhs who possessed substantial wealth in the form of livestock appeared to work harder than women in less well-off households and received less help from their spouses in managing the household. With respect to the treatment of male and female children, it appeared to me that Bedouin mothers disciplined (mostly with slaps on the hands or legs) daughters more frequently than sons, although I have no empirical evidence to support this impression.

Demographic data can provide an additional lens for assessing the valuation and treatment of women and girls. Gender disparities in early child mortality and morbidity are commonly used indicators of gender discrimination. Female infants are believed to have a biological advantage over male infants, possessing stronger immune responses, lower fatality rates from infections and respiratory conditions, and a lower likelihood of being born premature.[19] For these reasons, at low levels of early male mortality, females are expected to have about a 21 percent advantage over males in infant mortality and an 18 percent advantage over males in under-five mortality.[20] Tables 4.1 and 4.2 provide partial life table estimates of Bedouin mortality by gender. These estimates are taken from reproductive-history interviews conducted with 240 Bedouin women between the ages of fifteen and fifty-four in 2000–2001. Demographic estimates indicate that the female infant-mortality rate is .045 (table 4.1) and the male infant mortality is .060 (table 4.2). Infant mortality is more than 30 percent lower for females. Whereas infant mortality is lower for girls than boys, the opposite pattern is found for child mortality. Child mortality is .018 for females (table 4.1) and .015 for males (table 4.2). In terms of under-five mortality, approximately 93.78 percent of female children survive to age five. In other words, approximately 6.2 percent, or one in sixteen, of all Bedouin girls die before reaching the age of five. With respect to male under-five mortality, 92.59 percent of male children survive to age five. That is, approximately, 7.4 percent, or one in 14, of all Bedouin boys die before reaching the age of five. Bedouin girls are at a slight survival disadvantage over boys in the one to four age group—a pattern found in other Middle Eastern settings.

Higher mortality among female children ages one to four has been re-

Table 4.1. Mortality measures on ever born female children of 240 Bedouin women

Exact age[a]	Started Interval	Currently in Interval	Completed Interval	Deaths	q_x	l_x	d_x
0	681	38	643	29	.045	100,000	4,500
1	614	101	513	9	.018	95,500	1,719
5	504	163	341	0	.000	93,781	0
10	341	135	206	1	.005	93,781	469
15	205	99	106	1	.009	93,312	840
20	105	88	17	1	.059	92,472	5,456
30+	16	16	0	0		87,016	

Note: [a] The length of each interval is determined by the difference between age x and x+1, hence the first interval is one year in length; the second interval is four years long; the third through the fifth are five years long; the sixth interval is ten years long; and the final interval is open-ended.

Table 4.2. Mortality measures on ever born male children of 240 Bedouin women

Exact age[a]	Started Interval	Currently in Interval	Completed Interval	Deaths	q_x	l_x	d_x
0	718	38	680	41	.060	100,000	6,000
1	639	114	525	8	.015	94,000	1,410
5	517	150	367	3	.008	92,590	741
10	364	142	222	0	.000	91,849	0
15	222	108	114	1	.009	91,849	827
20	113	90	23	0	.000	91,022	0
30+	23	23	0	0		91,022	

Note: [a] The length of each interval is determined by the difference between age x and x+1, hence the first interval is one year in length; the second interval is four years long; the third through the fifth are five years long; the sixth interval is ten years long; and the final interval is open-ended.

ported in Jordan[21] and the Gulf countries of Qatar[22] and Kuwait,[23] but not in the United Arab Emirates.[24] Nevertheless, the same family-health surveys indicate that gender discrepancies in child mortality are not large. Reviews of demographic data on children in the Middle East and North Africa have uncovered numerous instances of excess female mortality in the one to four age group during the 1970s and 1980s as well as the 1990s; however, other indicators of child health (nutritional status, infections, and immunization) show a female advantage.[25] In virtually all Arab countries, infant mortality is higher than child mortality[26] and under-five mortality is higher for boys than girls.[27] Because the Lebanese and Syrian Maternal and Child Health Surveys do not provide gender-specific one to four mortality measures for the time period coterminous with the present study, it is not possible to determine whether the same pattern of slightly higher mortality among girls ages one to four is present in either country. The only evidence of gender disparity in child health in Lebanon and Syria lies in consultation for treatment of diarrhea and cough, and even here gender differences in morbidity are slight and tend to favor girls.[28] Bedouin mortality experiences shown in tables 4.1 and 4.2 can be compared to Ansley Coale and Paul Demeny's model life tables. It appears that the l_x calculated from the children born to 240 interviewed Bedouin women corresponds to the "West" models level nineteen, with an expectation of life at birth of sixty-five years for females and sixty-one years for males.[29] A cultural preference for sons in patriarchal societies can skew the sex ratio in favor of males. Natural sex ratios at birth in human societies are estimated to be close to 1.059 males/females. The Bedouin sex ratio at birth is 718/681 = 1.05 (see tables 4.1 and 4.2), which allows us to rule out sex-selective practices of infanticide or abortion.

When asked about the ideal gender composition for a Bedouin family, half of the women whom I interviewed stated that they preferred a gender-balanced family, with an equal number of boys and girls (120/240 = 50.0 percent). Slightly over one-fourth of Bedouin women indicated no gender preference (64/240 = 26.7 percent). Roughly one-fifth of women during reproductive-history interviews stated that they preferred a family with more sons than daughters (49/240 = 20.4 percent). The number of women who expressed a preference for more daughters than sons was small (7/240 = 2.9 percent). Aside from the fact that just over 75 percent of Bedouin women expressed a desire for a gender-balanced family configuration or no gender predilection, there is also a clear preference for large families among the older generation of Bedouin women (those 40 years and older in 2000). The fact that older cohorts prefer large family sizes points to the positive valuation of children and not an unmet need for contraception to limit births.

Large Families of Procreation

Reflexivity is implied in both social conduct and the discursive accounts of conduct. Discursive formulations of action can either be prompted by routine monitoring on the part of human actors or by questions emanating from others.[30] From ethnographic queries and conversations on the value of children, some of which were initiated by Bedouin actors themselves, I was able to identify three intersecting themes or narratives—economic, familial, and emotional—that capture some of the discursive formulations on the meaning of children. The identified themes overlap considerably and were often simultaneously invoked.

Bedouin women describe children as "partners in labor," who provide ongoing economic support and help take care of their parents in old age. Women and men discuss how when they are nearing "the end of their life," children will help care for them and support them. Having children guarantees that one will not want for anything and will not die alone. The most frequently proposed explanation for high fertility in the anthropological literature is the demand for labor—an explanation that flips Malthusianism on its head by arguing that children are a source of wealth, not misery. The economic benefits of children are usually delayed until children are old enough to provide economic assistance to their families, which in Bedouin communities usually occurs when the child reaches the age of eleven or twelve. Young households at the beginning of the family life cycle, with a higher proportion of consumers (young dependent children) relative to producers (workers), have a tougher time than those with older children who work and contribute to household expenditures. It is only relatively recently that the economic expenses of raising children have increased with the costs of schooling and the lost labor of children who attend school instead of assisting with household economic activities (see chapter 6 for a comparative discussion of the changing costs of children).

An oft-repeated expression by women is that "a house full of children is better than a house full of money." The economic narratives of mothers and fathers are as much emotional and kinship-centered as they are economic. Parents place enormous emphasis on the emotional companionship and happiness that children bring. A small family is viewed as being a lonely family. Conversely, a large family is strong, secure, and content. In addition to promoting the strength and vitality of the family, children help confer adult status in the community. Having children is an important rite of passage that allows adults to gain the respect of their peers as they assume parental responsibilities. The counsel of adults who have children is said to be heeded to a greater degree than that of adults who have yet to begin childbearing, allowing for fuller participation in the community. As one man said to me: "If you do not have children, people do not consult you or seek your advice on problems." Individuals who have not managed a household and raised children are considered less socially adept. Furthermore, adult men and women without children are sometimes said to be "thick-skinned," for they do not understand the sentiments—grief, joy, frustration, and love—that come from bearing and raising children. Both women and men describe the centrality of children in kinship-making. Children are frequently described by women as a "new family" that partners create themselves—one that provides a link to and break from their family of origin.

The family of procreation carries on and replaces the family of orientation. The Bedouin mother who gave birth to eighteen children (the largest family size in my sample)—sixteen of whom survived—was her parents' only surviving child. She had one younger brother who died before his first birthday, leaving her as the only child. Her husband, the son of her father's brother, is himself an only child. While their parents arranged the marriage, she explains that both she and her spouse consented to the match because they liked each other and wanted to build a family of procreation to compensate for their modest families of orientation. She was married at the age of fourteen (four years younger than the average age at first marriage among women) and her husband was only two years her senior (albeit nine years younger than the twenty-five-year average age at first marriage among men). It is widely acknowledged that children, especially sons, are needed for carrying on the family name and guaranteeing the continuity of the lineage in patrilineal societies. However, women through patriparallel-cousin marriage not only remain within the family but grow and strengthen the patriline. The responsibility of physically defending and protecting the family and broader kinship segments often falls to men. In the event of a dispute, it is considered advantageous to have more men than the opposing side. As Muḥammad, an elder Bedouin tribal shaykh, explains:

> There is a saying, "Count your men and arrive at water." If the water from a stream is fifty kilometers away and if you do not have men, then they will attack you and steal from you and kill you on the road. So count your men, see how many you have, and if they are many, then go find water—do not be afraid . . . In this way [by having children], the tribe grows.

The physical protection provided by men is necessary for securing resources for survival. There is a clear recognition of strength in numbers. A large family increases the number of political followers in a tribal community and helps tribal segments mount a better defense against potential foes. Large families exude vitality and strength. No one can put you down, so to speak, if you have a large family. By having the same number of children as other families, Bedouins maintain egalitarianism. Having slightly more children than other families can provide a sociopolitical advantage and allows individuals to resist the assertion of dominance from outside the family unit. Women also describe the benefits of large families. There is social comfort, glory, protection, vitality, and beauty in a large family. Women refer to the social pleasure of being encircled by one's children, grandchildren, and great grandchildren during social visits. A large family is a glorious sight—a spectacle to behold. Some women reflected on having to negotiate larger family sizes with husbands who wanted smaller ones. One woman, Sarsak, explains her reasons for wanting to continue childbearing even though her husband was eager to stop after their fourth child:

> Children "put away" [or protect] the house and the house puts away/ protects children. Children make you feel proud in front of other people. People will say [about your children] that they are the son of so-and-so. My husband wanted to stop after we had four children . . . He said, "We can provide our children with a good life and enjoy our life together; we can be happy with a small family," but I wanted more children. I wanted us to have many children so that we could have dominion over all other Arabs.

In addition to inspiring sentiments of pride and glory, children allow for the possibility of social aggrandizement. Social status is a matter of reputation and representation. Because a child is always identified as the son or daughter of X, the more children one has the greater the possibility that one is known. Both male and female children affirm the continuity of the family by preserving the memory of their parents after death.

At first, I was incredulous when Bedouin women told me that they did not experience hardship in childbearing and child-rearing. I assumed that it was culturally inappropriate or taboo to complain about children. I also incorrectly believed that if I waited long enough, I would begin to see evidence of women's discontent. Bedouin women with large families repeatedly mentioned that they did not endure great strain or hardship in bearing and raising children. Raising children is a community matter, and the assistance of elder siblings and extended family members within the village can be counted on. This does not mean that Bedouin women do not draw attention to the hard work they perform in Bedouin society. They do. I often heard women compare themselves to men when describing the nonchild-related labor activities they perform. Their active participation in the agropastoral economy is beyond question. The notion that numerous children pose a burden on women might make sense in societies where women's productive and reproductive roles conflict. Postreproductive women, when they were of reproductive age, would work with young infants tethered to them by a sling. In a few rare instances, women recounted solitary birthing while working the agricultural fields as day laborers.

It is also important to keep in mind that, in terms of pregnancy and delivery, Bedouins whom I encountered in 2000–2001 were not living in a premodern culture devoid of maternal- and child-health services. The following sociological snapshot captures contemporary views of sex, pregnancy, and childbearing in traditional societies:

> For most women, in most cultures, and throughout most periods of history, sexual pleasure, where possible, was intrinsically bound up with fear—of repetitive pregnancies, and therefore of death, given the substantial proportion of women who perished in childbirth and the very high rates of infant mortality which prevailed.[31]

Bedouin women in the Bekaa have access to skilled peasant midwifery. In reproductive histories, older women reported delivering their children at home with the assistance of a peasant midwife well-reputed in the Bekaa or with the help of an elder Bedouin woman with childbirth delivery experience. No matter how limited their access to health services in comparison to peasant women, most Bedouin women enjoy at least partial access to modern clinics and hospitals in the Bekaa. As a result, childbirth is not linked to a fear of death.

Large families for older couples were taken-for-granted aspects of social life. During a conversation I had in 2001, an elder male in the company of his wife and extended family asked me: "How would it hurt you if you had ten children surrounding you . . . five boys and five girls? How would it detract from your life?" I myself had already started to imagine the possibility and began to compose my response. However, his wife did not like the question, which surprised me since it was asked with gentleness and without hint of judgment. She proceeded to interject on my behalf: "Do you not see that she is a woman of education? She is delaying [childbearing] until she completes her education. I am sure that she and her husband will have children when the time is favorable." The desired family size most frequently reported among women forty and older in 2000 was ten children— five boys and five girls. Bedouins prefer a gender-balanced family. There is also a recognition among the older generation that younger couples desire fewer children, although Bedouin women under forty still prefer a gender-balanced family of two boys and two girls.

Bedouin discourses on reproduction among older couples point to a procreative power and glory in large families. Bertrand Russell has identified different forms of power, including traditional religious or magical power (priestly power), kingly power, naked power (marked by brute force), revolutionary power (e.g., the Reformation), economic power, power over opinion, and creeds as sources of power, arguing that love of power and glory is a chief characteristic of human social life and social change.[32] According to Russell, there is no ultimate form of power (e.g., economic) from which all other forms are derived. Russell's list is suggestive, but not exhaustive. There is also a need for thick descriptions of subsidiary forms of power that account for the dynamic varieties of local experience. While Russell distinguishes between power and glory, the development of the latter is preliminary. Russell writes: "Of the infinite desires of man, the chief are the desires for power and glory. These are not identical, though closely allied: the Prime Minister has more power than glory, the King has more glory than power."[33] The desire for glory is grounded in fame, admiration, and reputation. However, Russell argues that because the desire for glory and the desire for power involve similar pursuits, the two motives may, pragmatically, be considered one and the same. Giddens has also provided social theorists with a way of conceptualizing the exercise of power in human societies. According to Giddens, power is not itself a resource, but resources are vehicles through which power is put into action.[34] Giddens finds fault with certain strains of Marxism that focus on "allocative resources" to the exclusion of "authorization" as a resource. Whereas "authorization" refers to "capabilities which generate command over *persons*," "allocation" refers to "capabilities which generate command over *objects* or other material phenomena."[35] Giddens argues that these two types of resources are distinct and should not be collapsed into the same category.

The power and glory of a large Bedouin family does not merely reside in the economic advantages that children bring. In addition to conferring economic support as laborers (allocation)—a sort of built-in labor pool—children provide sociopolitical support as followers and built-in defense and protection from individuals and groups in social interaction (authorization) with opposing interests. Individual actors can thus mobilize allocative or authoritative resources in the generation of power/resistance. Procreative power involves the galvanization of both types of resources in the exercise of power. However, more than just enacting power, procreation sustains and strengthens community. Bedouin children provide companionship and enhance the feeling of communion with others. The language of power does not fully capture the meaning of children. Love and connection are affirmed through the experience of family-building. Children and families of procreation are the foundations of nurturing communities. The bearing and raising of children help build meaningful, supportive, and long-lasting communities. Given the importance of children in building economically and emotionally nurturing communities, one might suspect that married couples, particularly women, with few or no children might be at a social disadvantage. During my fieldwork in Bedouin communities, I came across only one infertile woman of postreproductive age (see below). The low level of primary sterility in Bedouin communities is not unexpected. After all, high Bedouin fertility, measured by the total fertility rate, is achieved by a combination of early weaning and marriage, low rates of marital dissolution, low levels of primary sterility, and low contraceptive use/effectiveness. Given that high fertility is the norm among older women born between 1942 and 1960 and that only 6.9 percent of these postreproductive women have family sizes of four and under (see table 2.2), what accounts for the lower fertility of these women? Do Bedouin women with fewer children in a high-fertility society face social stigma of any kind?

"Smaller" Families of Procreation

Couples with fewer children or no children often augment the size of their families through polygynous marriage. Bedouin women in polygynous marriages have lower fertility than women in monogamous marriages. Table 4.3 compares the average number of live births according to polygynous status. While only 9.8 percent of Bedouin women are in polygynous marriages, those women have almost three fewer children on average than women in nonpolygynous marriages. Polygyny can lower fertility through various social and biological mechanisms: higher divorce, age difference between spouses, postpartum abstinence, sterility of first wives, breastfeeding practices, disease transmission, and coital frequency. Among the Bekaa Bedouin, the lower fertility of polygynous couples is due to biological infertility or subfertility on the part of first wives. If we disaggregate first and second wives in polygynous marriages, we find that there is no significant difference in fertility between polygynous second wives and monogamous wives. However, polygynous first wives have significantly fewer live births than polygynous second wives *and* monogamous wives.

Misconceptions about polygyny and its social causes in Muslim Arab societies abound. The vast majority of Bedouin women are in monogamous

Table 4.3. Mean number of live births by polygynous status among 102 postreproductive Bedouin women

Marriage Type	No.	Mean Live Births
Polygynous	10	6.7 ± 3.7
Nonpolygynous/Monogamous	92	9.3 ± 2.6
Total	102	9.1 ± 2.9

marriages (90.2 percent). It is interesting to note that Bedouin women in monogamous marriages spoke very unfavorably about polygyny, whereas women actually in plural marriages did not voice the same negative sentiments about polygyny. Only one woman in my sample (whom I have identified by means of a pseudonym) was infertile. Shamsa's experience with polygyny and infertility helps illustrate how women confront and negotiate childlessness in conjunction with their spouses. Shamsa, her husband, and her senior co-wife are all patriparallel cousin relations. The impetus behind Shamsa's marriage as the second junior wife is a direct consequence of her senior co-wife's subfertility. The senior co-wife only bore two children: a daughter and a deaf son. As the second wife, Shamsa was even less successful at reproducing than her cousin co-wife. Shamsa became pregnant and delivered a stillborn child soon after her marriage. Complications during the delivery rendered her infertile. After a few years, Shamsa adopted her sister's daughter so that she would have an opportunity to experience motherhood. Shamsa herself recognizes the value of children: "A woman who has children is considered to have *marj'a* (recourse/refuge/shelter/sanctuary). No matter how much she and her husband get upset, she still has *marj'a*. She has a child in the house."

Ten and a half years into her marriage, Shamsa approached her husband, telling him that it was the appropriate time to take on yet another wife so as to grow the family. In recounting her conversations with her spouse, she explained that a woman who loves her husband would not want him to die without heirs. The Bekaa Bedouin do not practice sororal polygyny, but women are supposed to initiate the second marriage transaction (as this is considered the culturally appropriate practice); and in such cases, women tend to select a co-wife with whom they are close.[36] Shamsa had a younger kinswoman from the same tribe in mind for her husband. Yet, her partner expressed little interest in taking on a third wife, even if it implied building a large family; he was satisfied with his procreative family.

Normative rules surrounding polygyny provide important cultural safeguards for women. The normative expectation or requirement that first wives initiate second marriages is one example. During conversations about infertility, men in particular explained the importance of helping a childless woman overcome any sorrow she might feel as a result of being childless. A well-known Bedouin proverb recounted to me by several individuals states that a man whose wife is infertile must wait ten years before taking on another wife. The Old Testament contains a similar account of polygyny. If we use ethnography to read the Bible, the story of Abraham and his barren wife, Sarah, becomes intelligible as a story about infertility and polygynous marriage in a small-scale, tribal nomadic community. In Genesis, God says to Abraham: "I will make you a great nation; I will bless you and make your name great."[37] God said further: "Look now toward heaven, and count the stars, if you are able to number them." And He said unto him, "So shall your descendants be."[38] Yet, in spite of God's promises, Sarah remained infertile. As a result, Sarah enjoins Abraham to take her maid as a second wife, believing that he might obtain children by her. Ultimately, Abraham "heeded the voice of Sarai,"[39] agreeing to enter into a polygynous union. We are expressly told that this second marriage—facilitated by Sarah—was only entered into by Abraham ten years after his first wife was unable to bear children "Then Sarai, Abram's wife, took Hagar her maid, the Egyptian, and gave her to her husband Abram to be his wife, after Abram had dwelt ten years in the land of Canaan."[40]

Among Bedouin tribes in the Bekaa Valley today, there is a similar association between polygyny and infertility/subfertility. There is even a similar ten-year waiting period and cultural expectation that a wife will approach her husband and initiate the marriage process. Bedouin do not consider it appropriate for the male partner to initiate second unions or make overtures to a woman and express interest in her as a potential wife. Ideally, it is the first wife's role to approach, if not select, a potential second wife. (I myself was approached by a woman in a monogamous marriage who was trying to persuade me to become her junior co-wife. She praised her husband's good temperament and suggested that I would teach the children English while she would care for the sheep.) The emotional bond between husband and wife is not merely founded upon the woman's ability to bear children. Women are still valued for their labor, their social roles in the tribal community, and the emotional companionship they provide their partners. In spite of her status as a barren co-wife, Shamsa nevertheless holds a privileged position in her husband's affections. She describes the loving relationship between her and her spouse and how they have continued to eat together almost every day since the day they were first married. Polygynous unions, like other marriage practices, are interpreted, negotiated, and sometimes challenged by marital actors and other family members. Not all men adhere to social rules with regard to polygynous marriage. Some husbands, in conjunction with their partners, decide not to enter into second marriages at all, while other husbands (especially younger generations of Bedouin men) may initiate a second marriage without the cooperation of their first wife and before the ten-year waiting period.

Polygyny is an option available to monogamous couples who wish to compensate for their smaller families of procreation. However, not all cases of low fertility in the Bedouin population can be attributed to subfertility on the part of polygynous women. Smaller completed family sizes are also found among Bedouin women whose marriages were terminated by the death of their spouse. Marital disruption can be caused by either divorce or widowhood. Marriages are highly stable in Bedouin communities. The timing of marriage was found to have changed little among recent age cohorts of Bedouin women (see chapter 2). The average age at first marriage is the same for younger women (fifteen to thirty-nine in 2000) and older women (forty and over in 2000). The incidence of divorce among 102 postreproductive or near-postreproductive Bedouin women was only 2.9 percent.

Low divorce rates are a broader demographic feature of Arab societies, most of which experienced a decline in divorce over the course of the twentieth century. While researchers attribute higher divorce in the past to traditional Muslim law, which enabled men to easily obtain divorce,[41] such interpretations should be approached with caution, as the microhistorical dynamics involved in the stabilization of marriage are not well understood. It is possible that the decline in the divorce rate is linked to economic changes that increased the importance of the spousal bond and undermined women's broader kinship ties. Low rates of divorce have been reported in both Syria and Lebanon. In Syria, approximately 95 percent of first marriages were still intact at the time of a survey in 1993.[42] The proportion of Lebanese women whose first marriage was still intact at the time of a survey in 1996 was nearly 98 percent.[43] Separation is almost always preferred over divorce, although separation is poorly studied in both Syria and Lebanon.

In Bedouin communities of the Bekaa Valley, it is not unusual for women to leave their husbands and return to their parental home if they have a serious disagreement with their husbands. However, separations, and the cessation of sexual activity that often accompanies them, were not found to lower Bedouin fertility, as separations were usually of short duration. Similarly, divorce has little impact on fertility, as almost all Bedouin divorcées remarried within five years. The same cannot be said for widowhood. Bedouin widows did not remarry or wish to do so. Widowhood has a depressive effect on Bedouin fertility. Several Bedouin women, including the two women in table 2.2 with a completed family size of three, were widowed at a young age and chose not to remarry in spite of pressures and objections from family members, especially brothers and fathers. Women expressed concern that a new husband would not be as devoted to children from her previous marriage. Widows also cite affection for their deceased husbands as a main reason for not remarrying. Widows voiced a general desire to remain unmarried and manage their own household with the support of their children and extended family members.

Low fertility on the part of some postreproductive Bedouin women also raises the question of how women and their partners use contraception to regulate family size. I found no evidence to suggest that lower fertility on the part of some women could be attributed to contraceptive use. Bedouin women use traditional contraception for both spacing and late stopping. Postreproductive women with larger families reported using traditional contraception late in their reproductive lives to prevent further childbearing. However, one of my interlocutors reported using pills to abort her last three pregnancies (at roughly four months into each pregnancy) after the birth of her last child. The woman in question had a total of nine live births (although her second child did not survive). She was 17 years old when her first child was born and 32 years of age at the time of her last birth. She cited her health as a reason for not wanting further children and made her decision to end her last pregnancies independently, without consulting her spouse. This is an example of late stopping, which was common among postreproductive Bedouin mothers in my sample. However, the most commonly reported form of contraception was withdrawal, followed by breastfeeding. Withdrawal was reported more for spacing births apart during the early years of marriage, while breastfeeding was reported by older women to prevent further pregnancy.

Withdrawal has often been called the "male method" of contraception, because it requires male cooperation. Older Bedouin men take pride in their withdrawal skills, faulting younger husbands for lacking the sexual self-control believed to be necessary to practice withdrawal successfully. Withdrawal is usually described with euphemisms like "between me and him" or "throwing outside." Roughly 40 percent of postreproductive Bedouin women indicated that at some point in their reproductive lives, they used traditional contraception for spacing or late stopping. Yet, there is no evidence that traditional contraceptive use contributes to lower fertility among Bedouin women. Women who reported using contraception (mostly traditional contraception) actually had slightly higher fertility than those who did not, although the differences were small. This could be due to the fact that couples that report using withdrawal had better communication and more frequent sex (and thus slightly higher fertility). Either way, traditional contraceptive *use* does not necessarily imply *effectiveness*.

The frequency of sexual intercourse in marital relationships can also influence fertility, but coital frequency is notoriously difficult to measure. Bedouin women reported having regular sexual relations with their spouse—once or twice per week, on average. Women in *ghaṣb* or "forced" marriages expressed the most dissatisfaction with their intimate lives, at least early on in their marriages. Because there were only four forced marriages in my sample, it was not possible to determine if women in these unions had lower fertility. At least in the cases I found, there was no low-fertility pattern. In one instance, a forty-year-old Bedouin wife and mother of nine children was impelled to marry a friend of her father's. Initially, her brother wanted to arrange a sister-exchange marriage (in which men exchange sisters) when she was fourteen, but she refused the match. The family solicited the counsel of a well-respected Bedouin tribal shaykh from Syria to serve as an intermediary (between sister and brother) and bring about a resolution. She explained her dislike for her fiancé to the Bedouin shaykh, who was sympathetic to her situation and ultimately endorsed the termination of the engagement. Her success in refusing a sister-exchange union was somewhat muted by the fact that her father (whom she loved and respected) arranged the second match to one of his close friends—a man whom she did not know. She gave her consent to the marriage reluctantly. The woman in question, who chooses to remain unnamed, describes her initial physical aversion to her partner:

> When we got married, I refused for over a month to let him come near me and consummate the marriage. It was very hard [for me]. I do not know . . . I did not know him. He was a stranger [or nonrelative]. And how was he going to see my flesh bare? He was a stranger [to me] . . . It was [hard for me] because we were strangers and because there was no love. When there is love, he and I will feel that we love each other, but when there is no love it is very hard. But we 'got up' [i.e., rallied]. He treats me with tenderness and respect. I go to my family's. I go to my neighbors. I go to my friends, and he does not say to me, 'Where are you going?' He tells me to do whatever makes me comfortable.

Gender tensions are visible at the most intimate levels of experience. And yet stories of forced marriages do not turn out as tragically as one might assume. Women's defiance sets the stage for ongoing negotiations. Women do not surrender their autonomy within marriage. Marriage is something continually worked at by those who sustain it in their day-to-day conduct. Bedouin women's experiences of love and sex in marriage are not fixed and steady, but subject to fluctuations over time. Nevertheless, sexual frequency appears to vary less than sexual satisfaction. The period of postpartum sexual abstinence also varies, but most Bedouin women abstain from sex for at least forty days after giving birth. Either way, sexual frequency does not predict variation in fertility levels among Bedouin women.

Breastfeeding was the second most commonly reported traditional method of contraception used by women for spacing and late stopping. The contraceptive effects of breastfeeding are widely known among Bedouin women. Several mothers over forty reported breastfeeding their last child for a longer duration so as to avoid further pregnancy. The cessation of breastfeeding among most women occurs between thirteen and eighteen months. One of the most common reasons women gave for weaning (at earlier parities) was pregnancy. This is significant because it points to the unintended consequences of action. Women intended to wean their children later, but reported the interruption of breastfeeding by pregnancy. Bedouin women's workloads may interrupt on-demand feeding practices and its contraceptive advantages. Bedouin breastfeeding practices are more similar to those found in Syria than those found in Lebanon.[44] Short birth spacing is one of the main proximate determinants of high Bedouin fertility, but, conversely, the wider spacing of births can delay pregnancy and reduce infant and child mortality (see chapter 3). While breastfeeding duration is the most important predictor of birth-interval length, I was not able to ascertain a significant influence of breastfeeding duration on completed family size. The problem of recall bias could be a factor, as could the influence of other competing factors on the total number of children born. Other less frequently reported traditional methods of contraception designed to space births include drinking a henna/water mixture and ingesting raw green coffee beans (on the first day of a menstrual cycle for an entire year), although neither method is associated with lower fertility.

Conclusion

High fertility like that found among particular cohorts of Bedouin women is frequently diagnosed as symptomatic of Arab women's "inferior" and "subordinate" status. The population (bomb) threat is painted as a military threat that is ethnically (Arab) and religiously (Muslim) marked. From an imperialist frame, it is not only Arab women who need to be rescued from high fertility, but Western civilization itself. Embedded in these imperialist discourses on high fertility is the pseudofeminist language of "liberation." Colonial logics are Orwellian. Instead of calling for the colonial subjugation of Arab women, they dehumanize Arab men and call for the "liberation" of Arab women. Similarly, social-scientific accounts from a mainstream liberal frame often reinforce colonialism/imperialism. The agency of Third World women is usually undermined or dismissed, making it difficult to even imagine a social world where large families do not burden women and might actually be preferred by them.

Gender disparities in health and antifemale discrimination in Arab countries are frequently exaggerated. A gender bias in child mortality is discernable in Bekaa Bedouin communities and in several Arab countries, with girls ages one to four having slightly higher mortality than boys. However, overall, demographic actualities point to a lack of pronounced gender disparities in health in the contemporary Middle East. Greater attention is needed to the characteristic form and meaning of gender bias and how it varies across time and setting. It is important to examine the local meaning of childbearing in conjunction with the empirical occurrence of childbearing. Local Bedouin narratives on children help to make sense of high fertility and the social preference for large families. Attention to internal diversity in Bedouin family sizes and women's reproductive experiences shows that infertility and subfertility produce no-child and low-child families, respectively. Although rare, subfertility or infertility on the part of first wives is a common impetus behind polygynous marriage. Widowhood also contributes to lower female fertility, as marriage and childbearing are terminated by the death of a woman's spouse. Yet, unlike divorcées, Bedouin widows prefer not to remarry, which keeps their fertility down. The reluctance to remarry on the part of widows is largely due to concerns over the well-being of children from their first marriage. Bedouin discursive accounts point to the importance of placing childbearing and family formation in social context. Subjective accounts of the meaning of children are not mere abstractions but have contextual features. The next chapter places consanguineous marriage practices in political-economic and social context, demonstrating that close-kin marriage is an important social medium through which kinship and community are re-created.

5

Marriage between Kin

Making sense of close-kin marriage and its cultural meanings has long preoccupied anthropologists.[1] It is well known that patriparallel-cousin marriage (marriage between the children of brothers) is the culturally preferred marriage pattern in Middle Eastern societies. That is, the ideal marriage partner for a woman is her *ibn 'amm* (father's brother's son) or from the man's point of view his *bint 'amm* (father's brother's daughter). The specific question that I seek to address in this chapter is: why do the Bekaa Bedouin prefer marriages between close kin in general and patriparallel cousins in particular? In exploring indigenous experiences of marriage between relatives, I attempt to lay out the ways in which people reproduce and modify kinship structures, how kinship articulates with other social domains (marriage, gender, and occupation), and the linkages between biology and culture in the study of kinship. My main contention is that consanguineous marriage is more than a manifestation of Durkheimian social facts of kinship exercising constraints on individuals, but that by marrying relatives, individual agents reproduce those social kinship structures. Individuals do not uniformly or equally enter into patriparallel-cousin marriages, but do so depending on their occupation and other interests in society.

Consanguineous Marriage: Structure, Agency, and Meaning

The cultural preference for marriage between close kin is a salient feature of Bedouin matrimonial life. All societies have norms regulating marriage that place some form of constraint on women's and men's so-called choices. While analysts generally place consanguineous marriages under the category of arranged marriage, consanguineous unions sometimes reflect the preference of both marriage partners, raising questions about the prudence of drawing a sharp line between choice and constraint.[2] The most common form of consanguineous union worldwide is that between first cousins.[3] In the Middle East, marriage between parallel cousins, particularly patriparallel cousins, constitutes the predominant type of first-cousin union.

A recent review of national-level data from the Middle East shows that the frequency of first-cousin marriage (both cross and parallel forms) varies, ranging from a low of 15 percent in Turkey to a high of 41 percent in Saudi Arabia.[4] In looking at first marriages among 281 Bekaa Bedouin women born between 1942 and 1985, a substantial minority of them (45.2 percent) were found to be consanguineous (between second cousins or closer). First-cousin marriages (37.7 percent) account for over 80 percent of all consanguineous marriages, and patriparallel-cousin marriages (24.91 percent) comprise over 65 percent of all first-cousin marriages (see table 5.1). The high incidence of first-cousin marriage among the Bekaa Bedouin is comparable to that found among other marginal and traditionally nomadic peoples in the Middle East, such as the Bedouins of the Negev (40 percent) and Baluchis of southeastern Iran (44 percent). The highest rates of first-cousin marriage are found in countries (Saudi Arabia, Syria, and Qatar) with historically sizable nomadic populations.[5] In situations where geographic isolation, population dispersion, and mobility restrict mating opportunities, intermarriage between close kin could simply be a default marital strategy. Such a simple geographic explanation, however, is not without problems. Because nomadic movements coincide with the seasonal availability of resources, marriage exogamy could also make it easier for nomadic peoples, especially those living in precarious arid environments, to form a dispersed network of alliances over larger areas. These social networks can provide vital information about resource availability and make migrations smoother.[6]

Table 5.1. Prevalence of Bedouin consanguineous marriage

Consanguineous Marriage Type	No.	%
Patriparallel Cousin (FaBroSo)	70	24.91
Patricross Cousin (FaSiSo)	8	2.85
Matriparallel Cousin (MaSiSo)	15	5.34
Matricross Cousin (MaBroSo)	13	4.63
FaFaBroSo (first cousin once removed)	9	3.20
FaBroSoSo (first cousin once removed)	8	2.85
FaFaBroSoSo (second cousin)	4	1.42
Other	154	54.80
Total	281	100.00

Rather than being geographically imposed, reproductive isolation is more often self-imposed through cultural arrangements of mating and marriage. In order to explain the cultural preference for consanguineous marriage in settings where geographic isolation, small population size, and mobility are not constraining factors, social scientists frequently invoke economic explanations. Marriage within the family may help facilitate unions among the poor by allowing them to circumvent economic payments associated with marriage. Intrafamilial marriages can also be beneficial to wealthier segments of the population in as much as they prevent the fragmentation of agricultural property or patrimony[7] and loss of social status.[8] Whereas only a few of my Bedouin interlocutors indicated that first-cousin marriages are more economically viable since bride-price payments are sometimes lower for relatives, several respondents provided economic explanations for sister-exchange marriage (where two men marry each other's sisters). In the latter marriages, it is possible to avoid bride-price altogether. As 'Alī explains:

> He who has four or five sons has to pay money. Now, how much is the *mahr* (bride-price/indirect dowry)? Let's say you have five [unmarried] boys and you asked for my daughter [in marriage]. I need to take the money payment from you. We must agree on the money, you and I, . . . five hundred thousand, one million, two million [Lebanese pounds], and if you have a daughter and I have a daughter, [then] you take my daughter for your son, and my son takes your daughter. This would be better for you than to go pay money. And she [your daughter] will bring with her furnishings [mattress hand-stuffed with sheep wool]; she assembles her belongings [i.e., trousseau] for the house.

Marrying off sons can be expensive. In the context of large families, the economic difficulty in securing bride-price payments for sons is relaxed through sister-exchange marriage, which characterizes 12.8 percent of Bedouin marriages. High fertility and near universal marriage would be difficult to maintain without practices like sister-exchange marriage, which make getting married more affordable. Although economic explanations for sister-exchange marriage and consanguineous marriage may sound convincing, Bedouin women and men rarely offered economic rationalizations for the latter. There is also no evidence of a higher prevalence of consanguinity among poorer Bedouins or those with less inherited wealth (in the form of land, livestock, and machinery). However, rather than dismiss economic arguments altogether, I will revisit the issue at the end of the chapter, when I shift attention to the broader political-economic context of consanguineous marriage.

There is a general agreement among most scholars of the Middle East that marriage to a patriparallel cousin is a social expression and affirmation of kinship solidarity and a means of upholding the legitimacy of agnatic bonds.[9] Bedouin explanations for consanguinity in many ways parallel analytical interpretations. Abu Barakāt describes the importance of patriparallel-cousin marriage in upholding agnatic bonds:

> Outsiders, strangers, in the days of kings they cared about protecting their *mīrāt* (inheritance/patrimony/fortune), so they marry within the family to preserve their inheritance and not lose it. But Bedouins do not look to see if they have inheritance or do not have inheritance. The sons of your son are yours; the sons of your daughter are not. When your daughter is married to her *ibn ʿamm*, her son will stand beside your son. But when your daughter is married to a nonrelative, her son will stand against your son. They [Bedouin] emphasize this practice so that the men of the family stay united. As they say, "cows of the yard graze together in the yard."

Preserving the family fortune appears to have little bearing on patriparallel-cousin unions in land-poor Bedouin communities.[10] The primary purpose behind these marriages is not preserving wealth in the form of patrimony, but preserving sociopolitical connections between male agnates. Abu Barakāt helps us answer a key question: if "the sons of your son are yours," why should anyone care whom a man marries? After all, in a patrilineal society, presumably the sons of a man's son (as opposed to the sons of a man's daughter) are de facto members of his lineage by virtue of being descendants from the male line. The lineage can still grow strong in numbers when a man marries a stranger, as long as he produces children, especially sons, with that stranger. Why prevent women of the patriline from marrying out, since descent is not reckoned through them anyway? While there does appear to be slightly greater control exerted over the marriage actions of women than men, the marriage preference for patriparallel cousins is not gender-specific. For every woman who marries her cousin, there is a man who marries his cousin. A balanced sex ratio and low rates of polygyny produce no pronounced gender discrepancy. Both women and men acknowledge the cultural preference for marriage between patriparallel cousins. One of the reasons for social concern over the woman's marriage partner, alluded to by Abu Barakāt, is that marriage between a woman and her *ibn ʿamm* guarantees that her sons will be absorbed into the larger agnatic unit. A woman's male agnates can thus count on the support and loyalty of her children. Conversely, if a woman enters into a patrilineally exogamous marriage, her children will no longer belong to her father's or brother's lineage, but to her husband's. Patriparallel-cousin marriage serves to unite a woman's sons with the men of the lineage, augmenting its overall size and strength and preventing the emergence of potentially rival factions.

The Bekaa Bedouin generally acknowledge that marriage between the children of brothers not only promotes cohesion among the closest of male kin, it also enhances the bond between husband and wife. A middle-aged Bedouin woman describes the practice as follows:

> Your *ibn 'amm* takes away your worries [literally "the clouds"]. Your *ibn 'amm* will be compassionate, protect you, respect you, and support you because you are relatives. After all, your fathers are brothers.

In explaining the marriage practice, Bedouins emphasize that marriage to your *ibn 'amm* is preferable because of your distinctive relationship within the lineage system. You are not just affines but the closest of agnates. Patrilateral-parallel-cousin marriage upholds and strengthens the primacy of kinship bonds; and kinship bonds, in turn, augment marriage bonds. Bedouin women and men describe the heightened degree of support and familiarity that marks such relationships. Those who are both relatives and lovers are said to have greater compassion for one another and be more mindful of their marriage duties. One Bedouin man married to his *bint 'amm* recounted the tenderness with which his wife attended to him while he was ill, claiming that his wife would have been less compassionate if she were a nonrelative.

Since kinship bonds precede marriage bonds, one might be tempted to conclude that reinforcing agnatic bonds is the primary motivation behind these unions. Lila Abu-Lughod argues that patrilateral-parallel-cousin marriage is the culturally ideal marriage form, because it reflects the "tribal socio-structural model" organized on the basis of patrilineal descent. The marriage practice is preferred "because it follows the patrilineal principle, subsuming the marital bond under the prior and more legitimate bond of kinship."[11] Abu-Lughod's argument echoes that of Pierre Bourdieu, who describes patriparallel-cousin marriage as a "refusal to recognize the relationship of affinity for what it is."[12] In effect, both scholars posit that blood bonds trump marriage bonds. Marriage is largely conceived of as a political tool used to unite and expand descent groups. The notion that the marital bond is weak and given legitimacy by prior bonds of kinship reinforces the idea of marriage as a subsidiary social tie.

My analysis is a slight revision of Abu-Lughod's and Bourdieu's thesis in as much as I argue that marriage is not a weak bond subsumed under kinship, but rather that marriage to (culturally recognized) kin helps reproduce kinship bonds. Marriage is not simply strong or stronger because it is based on kinship, but kinship is strong or stronger because it is based on marriage. Marriage reproduces the kinship system itself. I suggest that marriage between relatives re-creates *qarāba* or "closeness" and that marriage between strangers can create strangeness. While patriparallel cousins of the opposite sex are already bound to each other by relations of descent, marriage instantiates and gives meaning to those patrilineal bonds. Marriage helps keep those "significant affiliations significant."[13] The practice of patriparallel-cousin marriage in effect turns agnates into affines into close agnates. The failure to marry close kin can undermine or threaten bonds of kinship. Instead of proclaiming that kinship bonds are prioritized over marriage bonds in Bedouin Arab society, it would be more accurate to state that kinship bonds rely on consanguineous marriage bonds for their social reproduction. Without socially enforcing marriage to particular categories of kin, kinship itself is potentially violated. Kinship needs and depends on marriage to be reproduced from generation to generation. Marriage between those defined as "close" helps perpetuate kinship. Kinship based on genealogical ties is not a guarantee of *qarāba*, for kinship must be instantiated and reconstituted through social practices, including intrafamilial marriage. Patrilineal kinship is not conferred upon a man's descendants in perfunctory fashion. Kinship has always rested on a distinction between the biological and the social.[14] Bedouin kinship bonds rest on socially recognized biological relationships, but those bonds are not automatic. In other words, "Kinship is not a preexisting thing, but rather is something 'congealed.'"[15] Kinship is created, negotiated, instantiated in practice, and, therefore, malleable. Kinship bonds in Bedouin society must be activated and strengthened through reciprocal visiting, attending to ritual and ceremonial obligations, food sharing, and endogamous marriage. Marriage to strangers can weaken kinship.

Failure to adhere to expected social kinship norms results in social consequences, sometimes severe. In Emile Durkheim's view, it is society, not biology, that is coercive. Social facts constrain individual behavior. As Durkheim states:

> These types of conduct or thought are not only external to the individual but are, moreover, endowed with coercive power, by virtue of

which they impose themselves upon him, independent of his individual will. Of course, when I fully consent and conform to them, this constraint is felt only slightly, if at all, and is therefore unnecessary. But it is, nonetheless, an intrinsic characteristic of these facts, the proof thereof being that it asserts itself as soon as I attempt to resist it.[16]

Kinship beliefs and practices, like other social facts, are coercive; and the rejection of those rules and guidelines is often met with negative social sanctions. Bedouin couples that elope (almost always with distant kin or nonkin) must bear the consequences of social-norm violation as it pertains to marriage. In one instance, a Bedouin woman was shunned by her natal family for seven years because she secretly eloped with a nonrelative. In a similar case, a Bedouin woman, now in her early fifties, has yet to reconcile with her family over the fallout from her elopement, which occurred thirty years prior. During the interim, her mother passed away, frustrating hopes of reconciliation. One of my younger informants, in her mid-twenties, recounted a more recent incident in which her father's brother's son was so upset by her (and her parents') refusal of his marriage proposal that, weeks before her wedding to another man, he, in the company of his father, fired surprise shots at their house, nearly wounding members of her immediate family. The two brothers and their families have not spoken in the five years since the incident.

While it is clear that consanguineous marriage reflects constraints of the sociotribal structure in a Durkheimian sense, it does more than just represent that structure; it reproduces the kinship system itself. Marriage is an important means of forging kinship. Kinship is reproduced or transformed by the actions of social participants. Anthony Giddens has rejected the functionalist (Durkheimian) notion of homeostasis, in which a change in one item produces a sequence of events affecting others, so that the system *inevitably* returns to its original state. To say that social systems are "self-regulating" through feedback is not the same as saying that they are homeostatic. Feedback mechanisms can give rise to stasis, but they can also spur directional change via the selective screening or "filtering" of information. Giddens refers to the double character of structure as the "duality of structure," meaning that structure is not simply restraining of human agency but enabling as well.[17] Giddens' structurationist view highlights one of the weaknesses with the Durkheimian notion of structure—its failure to recognize that participants apply norms and rules drawn from the social order, but, in doing so, reconstitute that order.

Kinship structures should not be seen as either closed or fixed. Kinship can be undermined by failing to adhere to practices congruent with those roles. Just as an American biological father can become a "deadbeat dad," a Bedouin patrilineal relative can become a "stranger." Genealogy or biology is a necessary but not sufficient cause of closeness. One of the most important forms of kinship-making among the Bedouin is the practice of patriparallel-cousin marriage. This is borne out in Bedouin explanations of consanguineous marriage. As 'Abd al-Karīm, who is married to his father's sister's daughter, explains:

> Al-Badawī (A Bedouin) does not marry a stranger. If I marry *bint 'ammī* (my father's brother's daughter), then *ibn 'ammī* (my father's brother's son) will feel that 'my house is his house' . . . but if I marry a stranger, I would feel that my own mother is a stranger in my house. Whenever my mother came over, if my wife were a nonrelative . . . whenever my mother came to my house, I would feel like she is a stranger, based on my wife. My relatives would feel like strangers in my house. They would not act freely, which is the difference between marrying a relative and marrying a stranger.
>
> If I were to marry *bint 'ammī* or *bint 'ammtī* (my father's sister's daughter), then my aunts [father's brother's sisters] would come visit . . . if my cousin wife were destitute or dispossessed [literally "naked"], I would cover her [and] protect her. I would feel compassion for her; I would guard her honor and would not allow society to bask in [or gloat over] her misfortune and grief. If I were to marry a stranger, the environment would be altogether different—the household environment would be in disorder. This does not just apply to the Bedouin but all people. The prophet, peace be upon him, said: "Do not play around with *al-nasab* (consanguinity/lineage/kinship/ancestry/genealogy)." You cannot play with *nasab*. Take me for instance. I am Lebanese and [Bedouin] Arab; I could not marry a German, American, or Brazilian woman [pause]; someone from a different tribe, yes, maybe, but I could not bring a stranger into my house.

Marriage to nonkin creates social and emotional distance that can undermine patrilineal kinship bonds. By bringing a stranger into the house, close patrilineal relatives can become foreign, distant, and awkward in each other's company. They lose feelings of intimacy and relatedness. Marriage to patriparallel cousins preserves closeness between a man and his wider kin group, particularly in the social space of the home. The home is not simply a private space for the couple but an intersubjective space for welcoming visitors and bestowing hospitality, especially toward kin. 'Abd al-Karīm's response signals some flexibility in the delimitation of kinship. Close relatives within the tribal patriline are preferable, but other kin, including the father's sister's children, are not excluded as marriage partners. Marriage to an individual from a different tribe is not entirely out of the question either, as most Bedouin recognize the existence of a shared genealogical connection between different Bedouin tribes. Close-kin marriage helps to maintain and perpetuate kinship ties. Even mothers can become strangers to their children (the son/groom in this case) if they marry nonrelatives. The bond between husband and wife is recognized as an intimate bond. It is the wife who, by virtue of her kinship status, either reproduces intimacy and unites family members or creates distance and weakens blood ties. By marrying his patriparallel cousin, a man preserves and augments kinship bonds. He ensures that his male patriparallel cousins and other relatives will feel at ease in his home. Having related spouses in the house prevents it from falling into disarray and confusion. Social confusion and disorder arise when relatives become strangers as a result of marriage to strangers. Thus, affinity emerges as neither weak nor insignificant. It is the marital bond and procreation that help reproduce kinship bonds. There is even an antiquity and religious sanctity attached to the social practice, as the prophet Muḥammad's teachings on descent are invoked.

An interesting religious parallel can be found in the biblical story of Abraham and Sarah. Abraham, the first patriarch, through whom all three major religious traditions trace their descent, is commanded by God in the Old Testament to sacrifice his son Isaac, "Take now your son, your only son Isaac, whom you love, and go to the land of Moriah, and offer him there for a burnt offering on one of the mountains of which I shall tell you."[18] However, Abraham had already fathered his firstborn son, Ishmael, with his Egyptian handmaid, Hagar. It was his barren first wife, Sarah, who enjoined him to take her maid to produce a son. Sarah only later becomes pregnant and conceives Isaac. Although Ishmael is Abraham's eldest son, there is no real acknowledgement of love between Abraham and Ishmael in the book of Genesis. Indeed, Ishmael's very kinship status as Abraham's son is dismissed by God, who tells him, "In Isaac your seed shall be called."[19] Carol Delaney describes this denial of his firstborn son as an act of violence and exclusion:

Not only is Ishmael banished into the wilderness but he is also excluded from any inheritance. Then when God said to Abraham, "Take your son, your only son," Abraham did not contradict him and say, "But I have two sons." When God added, "whom you love," Abraham didn't proclaim, "But I love both." Out of sight, out of mind, Ishmael has vanished."[20]

Abraham's revocation of kinship to Ishmael is not so puzzling if we recognize the importance of the wife's consanguineous status in determining kinship bonds among Old Testament tribes. While rabbinic sources differ in their assignations of Sarah's kinship status, describing her as half-sister, niece, or patriparallel cousin,[21] they all regard her as close kin. Hagar is foreign, so Ishmael is foreign. Even though Ishmael shares half of Abraham's genetic material, Abraham fails to forge an authentic kinship with and compassion for Ishmael. Isaac is his "real" son, his only son whose mother shares a recognized kinship relation to the father. The marital relationship determines the authenticity of the father-son relationship.

The importance of bodily substance, especially "blood" (*dam*), for creating closeness or kinship among Bedouin family members is clear. As Layla, a Bedouin woman in her early thirties, explains:

> Their children [patriparallel cousins'] stay close to each other. They do not come from strange blood; they come from the blood of their kin—their mother, father, mother's sisters, father's brothers. A girl is for her patriparallel cousin. He holds onto her.

Patriparallel marriages help create and perpetuate kinship. Having blood in common is thought to make the bond between children stronger. Kinship requires marriage between kin so as to ensure that children are born close and "of the same blood." Children who share the same blood stay united and do not become strange. "Closeness" requires more than simple sexual procreation or being born to the same biological mother or father. To be truly close, children should be the product of marriage between socially recognized blood relatives. Brother and sister who are son and daughter of patriparallel cousin-spouses qualify as close siblings. Authentic kinship requires a culturally valued kind of biogenetic connection. Kinship requires the assistance of marriage. Biology requires the assistance of culture.

It is important to appreciate the multiple etiologies of blood as they pertain to kinship and kinship-making. Blood is not only an index of relatedness but of sentimentality and spatial proximity. Sarsak explains the importance of shared geography and sentimentality as they pertain to marriage between patriparallel cousins:

Your *ibn 'amm* is better; he is good. That is, he covers them [his female patriparallel cousins]; she does not become foreign; she does not go far; and he remains more tenderhearted than nonkin. Your *ibn 'amm* stays more compassionate in his heart toward her [his *bint 'amm*, or father's brother's daughter] than a nonrelative. That is, we leave her with her family, so if he sends her away [or] if he wrongs or oppresses her, [then at least] this one is her *ibn 'amm*.

By marrying her patriparallel cousin, a woman reaffirms familial bonds. She does not become foreign or distant—a stranger in effect—by marrying nonkin. Kinship is defined on the basis of both social and spatial proximity. To keep women "close" requires marrying within the family. A bride's natal family members are thus in a better position genealogically and geographically to look out for her and check male-on-female oppression. By marrying a stranger and moving away, kinship bonds are loosened. There is an important nurturing element here, as living close by and visiting create kinship. Mothers whose daughters married nonkin frequently complained that their daughter's husbands were less amenable to bringing them back home for social visits. Geographic distance creates social and emotional distance. By marrying outside of her kin group, a woman moves away and becomes distant and strange. As mentioned previously, patrilocality poses a particular problem for women. Women are protected by consanguineous marriage because residential proximity means that family members can influence and keep an eye on husbands.

Patriparallel-cousin marriage is itself a circumvention of female submission to patrilocality. Molly Levine describes how in Greek tradition "Penelope was the first woman to abandon father for husband in patrilocal marriage" and veiled as a result of her shame over this "betrayal"—the Greek version of a wife's "original sin."[22] Numerous Greek stories recount woman's desertion of father for husband or "repudiating the bond with the father."[23] Yet, patriparallel-cousin marriage obviates the bride's separation from her father and his lineage. Consanguineous marriage is considered socially preferable since it allows for a smooth adjustment of the wife to new relationships created through marriage.[24] Marriages that build on preexisting patrilineal bonds of kinship are particularly beneficial to women in patrilocal societies, like that of the Bedouin, since women are able to marry without losing ties to their natal family. However, more than just not betraying the patrilineal principle, women are central to its maintenance. Women are needed to authenticate patrilineal kinship bonds.

Kinship and gender are mutually constituted in the study of Bedouin

consanguineous marriage. As kinship is predicated upon marriage to socially recognized women relatives, gender emerges as a crucial component
of kinship-making. It would be inaccurate to suggest that intrafamilial marriage benefits men at the expense of women.[25] Patrilineally endogamous
marriages provide important social and emotional benefits to women. Both
women and men point to the protections and benefits afforded women by
close-kin marriages—benefits that relate to emotional comfort, economic
assistance, and physical protection. Women and men speak of deep sympathy, familiarity, and comfort between relative spouses. Feelings of em-
pathy between close paternal kin are said to enhance a man's respect for
his cousin-wife. Sarsak describes the heartfelt affection felt by a man for
his father's brother's daughter. Men are less likely to be harsh or oppressive
toward women who are members of their lineage.

By drawing upon genealogical ties, close-kin marriages provide a sort of
buffer against ill treatment of women. Rḥayla describes men's sympathy and
tenderness for their patriparallel cousin wives in poetic form:

> Her *ibn ʿamm* will not be hard on her.
> If he were to hit her, he would be hitting himself.
> If he were to speak [ill] of her he would be speaking [ill] of himself.
> Blood keeps the whole family close to one another.
> The children of strangers remain strange.

The identification of a man with his cousin-wife suggests an intersubjective
understanding of the self. There is a congruity, mutuality, and symmetry between spouses, united by descent and marriage. Consanguineous marriage
helps narrow the gap between husband and wife. The tension and potential
for violence is checked. Marriage and procreation between two related individuals also unites the wider kin group. The bond between couples, children, and family members is, in part, predicated on blood marriages. It is
widely acknowledged among Bedouin women and men that while patriparallel-cousin marriage affords special protections for women, marriage
to other patrilineal relatives can provide similar benefits. As one Bedouin
tribal shaykh explains:

> This [i.e., *ibn ʿamm*, or patriparallel-cousin marriage] is all because of
> the protectiveness of the bride's family toward their daughter. I would
> not want to give my daughter in marriage to a man who will use her
> for his own pleasure. It would be preferable to give her to her *ibn ʿamm*.
> If that is not possible, then the son of her *ibn ʿamm*, after that a mem-
> ber of her tribe, and so on . . . steps.

The marriage protections for women are linked to kinship at different levels of human social organization, but the principle is one of agnation. While emotional sympathies are believed to be strongest between patriparallel cousins, they extend to more distant paternal kin as well. Marriages between close paternal relatives other than patriparallel cousins constitute 7.47 percent of marriages (table 5.1). Yet, 89 percent of all couples (249/281) belong to the same tribe, affirming the broader centrality of agnation.

The emotional sympathies inscribed in patrilineal kinship are also partially extended to maternal relatives. Skūt affirms:

A mother would like for her daughter to marry her sister's son or her brother's son, so that he [i.e., the husband] is not hard on her like a stranger. She would like to give her daughter [in marriage] to *ibn silfa* (the son of her husband's brother) if he [i.e., her husband's brother] is married to her sister. A mother-in-law [in this situation] would not be hard on her daughter-in-law, because she would be her sister's daughter. There is deep sympathy between them.

Matrilineal kin are bestowed with similar feelings of mercy and compassion. A mother is eager for her daughter to marry her sister's son. Her husband's brother's son would also constitute a desirable match for her daughter, especially if the husband's brother in question were married to her sister. The motivation behind these matrilateral marriages is similar to those behind patrilateral marriages. Closely related to the concern of protecting a woman from her husband is that of protecting a woman from her mother-in-law. A mother-in-law who is also the maternal aunt of the bride is believed to possess greater tenderness toward her daughter-in-law because of their shared, uterine, kinship connection. Matriparallel-cousin marriage is the second most common type of first-cousin marriage in Bekaa Bedouin communities. Only two couples in my sample were double first cousins, related as both patriparallel and matriparallel cousins—in other words, the cousin couples in question were the children of brothers whose wives were also sisters. Anthropologists have described marriage between parallel cousins, both patrilateral[26] and matrilateral,[27] as a marriage between equals, given that the sibling parents of cousin spouses are of the same sex and presumably of similar status within the lineage. Brothers are considered social equivalents, as are sisters; thus, parallel marriages reflect marriage between "equals." The two most common forms of first-cousin marriage among the Bekaa Bedouin are those between the children of brothers (patriparallel) and the children of sisters (matriparallel) (see table 5.1). Marriage may help maintain social equality through the union between social "likes."

While some of the benefits behind consanguinity are gender-specific, other benefits appear to reflect the interests of both women and men. Blood is an index of familiarity, which can help prevent unpleasant surprises in marriage. Marriage between relatives, like marriage between friends, presupposes familiarity, thereby lowering some of the risks and uncertainties associated with marriage. One woman, who prefers to remain anonymous, articulates the importance of social familiarity:

> Bedouin prefer to take from [i.e., marry] each other. They do not like nonkin, because nonkin, they know nothing about them. They know nothing about the person and if he has, Allāh forbid, an enemy or a disease; they do not know ... When the person is a relative they know everything about them. Those who take from each other stay protective of their lineage/ancestry; that is, they are of good parentage or descent—they [the husband and wife] have taken from each other. They marry from each other so that their children stay from each other.

A close woman relative of hers added:

> We care about *aṣl* (descent/lineage/ancestry/parentage)—that his *aṣl* is good and that he is from a good family, not a thief or a scoundrel ... but someone who possesses *raḥma* (mercy/leniency/clemency/compassion/pity) and *shafaqa* (caring/pity/compassion/deep sympathy/humanity/mercy feeling/tenderness/kindness) . . . We know his grandfather and the grandfather of his grandfather. We know that he is a descendant of so-and-so, down to his father. He is of good descent.

Aṣl, which is often used interchangeably with "blood," refers to ancestry or origin, in a narrower sense, but, in a broader sense, encompasses a constellation of individual and interindividual attributes denoting reputation, character, intimacy, and familiarity. Blood is more of a metaphysical than a physical substance. Knowledge of a person's family background, genealogy, and social reputation are a testimony to one's emotional makeup, moral conduct, and health.[28] Evidence of honesty, trustworthiness, or virtue, and, conversely, of dishonesty, lechery, or vice is to be found in oral genealogical accounts. Information about an individual's physical and mental health can also be imparted through genealogies. A Bedouin woman in her late fifties noted that Bedouin strongly disapprove of marriage to a leper or to the descendant of a person afflicted with leprosy (*baraṣ*). Although the disease is not hereditary, it has a long incubation period with signs and symptoms appearing only after several years, making it a seemingly hereditary disease. Thus, blood descendants are preferable from a social and biological standpoint because they are known; they are an open book. A stranger, on the other hand, is, as one Bedouin man put it, "a 'closed watermelon'—no one knows what is inside."

In exploring the multiple etiologies of marriage between relatives, particularly patriparallel cousins, I have argued that blood or kinship symbolically encodes information—solidarity, compassion, spatial proximity, equality, familiarity, and health—linked to an identification with ancestry cohered through consanguineous marriage and procreation. Patriparallel-cousin marriage cements alliances among patrilineal relatives and prevents the rupture of kinship bonds between a woman and her lineage upon her marriage. Referring to such a descent system as "patrilineal" obscures the system's dependence on marriage and women. Patrilineality in this context requires the fusion of male and female lines of ascent. Even in Arab societies where the reckoning of descent is unilineal, there remains significant flexibility in systems of affiliation and marriage. Individual women and men draw upon the kinship structures of the society to which they belong and apply them through social praxis, thereby modifying or perpetuating those structures. Consanguineous marriage works to both exemplify and produce kinship. Marriage is not merely "a glue that holds two kin groups together"[29] but the water that helps patrilineal kinship bonds bloom. Affinal ties cannot be brushed aside as insignificant, given that kinship is re-created through marriage, especially (but not exclusively) marriage to a woman agnate.

The Political-Economic Context of Consanguineous Marriage

Within Bedouin society, the consanguineous-marriage actions of individuals reproduce kinship at the same time that kinship constrains the marriage practices of those individuals. However, not only are there different types of constraint that narrow the range of marriage options open to individual agents, but those constraints are historically shifting. Macro-level economic changes accompanying modernization create new contexts for marriage and kinship behavior. Marriage ultimately finds expression in particular social worlds and political-economic realities. It is also important to keep in mind that social constraints are not wholly determinative, but "enabling as well as constraining."[30] Individual agents do not uniformly or mechanically reproduce social structures. Rather, individuals interpret and act upon marriage sanctions or norms differently, depending on their divergent and opposing interests in society. It is in and through their actions that individuals facilitate the continuation, transformation, or rejection of social structures.

Table 5.2. Prevalence of Bedouin consanguineous marriage by occupation

Consanguineous Marriage Status	Occupation			
	Pastoralism	Sharecropping	Wage Labor	Other
First Cousins	35	48	20	3
Nonfirst Cousins	36	66	62	11
Total	71	114	82	14

Note: Pearson Chi-Square = 12.767 (df = 3, N = 281), p = .005.

If we look at the distribution of Bedouin consanguineous marriages shown in table 5.1 by occupation, we see clear distinctions. Table 5.2 shows that individuals involved in wage labor and related forms of employment are less likely to enter into consanguineous marriages. Approximately 49 percent of pastoralist couples are first cousins, compared to 42 percent of sharecroppers, 24 percent of wage laborers (agricultural and manufacturing), and 20 percent of couples involved in other/miscellaneous rural service and retail trade occupations (milkmen, butchers, truckers, cement masons, small grocers, and petty traders). From a purely economic standpoint, such a pattern may seem surprising. As mentioned previously, wage laborers who lack ownership of the means of production would appear to benefit from entering into low-cost consanguineous marriages. Neither is it true that pastoralists who enjoy greater productive wealth than all the other occupational groups are marrying close kin so as to preserve their wealth or elite social status. If that were the case, then we would expect the children of pastoralists only to marry the children of other pastoralists. The economic transition from pastoralist to peasant farmer and from pastoralist to proletariat is historically very recent (see chapter 2) and helps to explain the lack of occupational endogamy. Occupational designations refer to the dominant mode of production since marriage. Many wage laborers today were pastoralists in the not-too-distant past. In fact, most wage laborers were born to parents who worked as pastoralists a generation ago. It does not appear that productive wealth per se accounts for variation in the frequency of close-kin marriage between the occupational groups. In fact, there are no significant differences in productive wealth between sharecroppers and those in the other/miscellaneous occupational category (the latter actually have slightly greater productive wealth) and yet there are clear differences in the frequency of close-kin marriages between the two groups. Occupational groups also do not appear to represent clear-cut classes based on exploit-ative relations, but rather represent different local modes of production with somewhat distinct micro-level social relations and forces of production.

By considering the role of the family in production, we can make sense of the occupational differences in first-cousin marriage shown in table 5.2. If we recall from chapter 2, a major change in the Bedouin social economy oc-curred in the 1960s as camels were replaced with pickup trucks. The mech-anization of transport was part of a broader nexus of rapid modernizing forces, which David Harvey glosses as "time-space compression."[31] Trucks greatly reduced nomadic movements between winter and spring pastures. Migrations that once took weeks or months to complete now took hours or days. As Bedouin families remained in the Bekaa for longer periods of time, they developed closer economic ties to peasant society, hiring out their la-bor and renting their trucks to neighboring towns and villages. Between the 1960s and 1980s, families began selling a portion (and in some cases all) of their herds in order to purchase land and build homes for residence. Most Bedouin villages were founded by brothers or male agnates and thus largely consist of close kin. Kin cooperated closely in their herding activities and migrated together as a unit. As Bedouins became alienated from their herds, they accelerated their involvement in sharecropping, as well as agricultural and manufacturing wage labor. Hence, within the span of a few decades, we see that Bedouin have replaced their camels with trucks, built homes, estab-lished villages and mosques, placed some of their children in school, tran-sitioned away from a pastoral economy, experienced the epidemiological transition as well as the onset of fertility decline, and become participants in consumer capitalist culture.

Rural industrialization and growth of a new wage economy appear to have undermined the need for family members within the minimal agnatic unit to work together, as work roles have become increasingly individual-ized. Agricultural and manufacturing wage earners depend on the market value of their labor in a competitive economy. In short, as wage labor in-creases, the extended family ceases to be a unit of economic production, which may, in turn, lessen inducements behind intrafamilial marriage. Family cooperation in labor is more central to pastoralism and agricultural sharecropping than it is to wage labor or to specialized and individualized rural trade occupations. Marital relationships based on kinship consider-ations may decline as the family becomes more dependent on the market than the extended family.

Peasantization and proletarianization processes associated with capital-

ist development and state encapsulation also usher in new social relationships and institutional-spatial configurations. While the *sahel* and the farm
are more familiar socioecological environments, the mosque, the factory,
the school, the peer group, and the permanent village are relatively newer
spaces for Bedouin social interaction. For example, a young wage laborer in
her early twenties who has been married for five years recounted to me how
she met her husband at work—a food-processing plant, where both were
employed in assembly-line production. Socialization is being carried out by
individuals who are not part of the kinship network, which may change the
social criteria used in mate selection. Marriage reflects the realities of one's
socioeconomic environment. In terms of negotiating marriages, parents often support having children meet up in these new settings (i.e., work and
school, but particularly at school), provided that they follow culturally appropriate guidelines of honor and modesty. In the above example, the young
couple were not first cousins; however, they were both Bedouin and members of the same tribe. Perhaps, in the future, shared tribal affiliation will be
less important and a greater proportion of Bedouins will marry outside of
their tribe. With a greater emphasis being placed on organized religion, we
might also see an increase in Bedouin-peasant marriages.

Because estimates of the prevalence of consanguineous marriage are not
available for younger Bedouin women (more recent cohorts, born after
1985), the prediction that diversification and modernization of the Bedouin
economy will bring about a future decline in consanguineous unions remains unconfirmed. However, on my return fieldwork visit in 2007, I was
struck by how the five newly married Bedouin couples with whom I spoke
articulated the shifting emphasis from consanguineous marriages to individually chosen love marriages—a shift that reflects changes in the organization of daily life, the political economy, and changing demographics.
The impact of demographic transition on marriage is particularly relevant.
As fertility continues to decline and the size of the family shrinks in modern societies, the spousal bond is expected to become a more central locus
for intimacy and companionship.[32] The decline in infant mortality and increase in adult life expectancy means that couples can expect to spend a
greater portion of their lives together after their children marry and establish households of their own.

The increasing emphasis on love is not a sharp break with the past. At
least one-third of all Bedouin marriages are love or companionate marriages. Although fewer first cousins marry out of love, consanguineous marriage and companionate marriage are not mutually exclusive. In my sample,
at least thirteen women (13/106 = 12 percent) in first-cousin marriages and

seventy-seven women (77/175 = 44 percent) in nonfirst-cousin marriages indicated that they chose their partners and married on the basis of love and affection. Only four women in the entire sample (4/281 = 1 percent) reported being forced into marriage,[33] either by their parents or brothers. One Bedouin mother, whom I originally interviewed in 2000, was particularly strident in extolling the virtues of love marriages when we met again in 2007. Both of her daughters had recently wedded their patriparallel cousins. She praised the choices of both daughters, explaining how they socialized with their cousins at school and made their decisions on the basis of love. Younger women and men appear to have greater individual control over their marriage destinies.

Parallel to the growing emphasis on companionate marriage is a new kind of relationship being forged between love and commodity exchange; it's what Eva Illouz refers to as "the romanticization of commodities and the commodification of romance."[34] Courtship, engagement, and marriage are dependent on consumption. It is now customary, in the older Bedouin villages, for a Bedouin woman's fiancé to visit her at her family's house and invite her and other close kin to a restaurant for lunch. Courtship among the young involves buying appropriate clothing, accessories, and cosmetic products for social outings. Young Bedouin women dress in colorful Islamic-style clothing usually accompanied by head scarves, while young men wear more Western-style clothing—jeans, T-shirts or dress shirts. Reading of the opening verses of the Qur'an and signing of the wedding contract usually take place at the engagement ceremony. On the wedding day, the bridegroom comes for the bride in an expensive rental car. Ornate photo albums full of studio pictures documenting the engagement and wedding are increasingly commonplace, as are professional wedding videos. Consumer demonstrations of love parallel trends observed elsewhere (e.g., Spain,[35] Mexico,[36] and Iran[37]) of commodities increasingly defining intimate relationships.

Yet, for Bedouin in the Bekaa Valley, the most important consumer activities relate to building and furnishing the couple's new home for marriage. Aside from running water and a water heater for the bathroom and basic household appliances (refrigerator and washing machine), the average Bedouin home now includes bed linens and furniture (dresser and mirror) for the bedroom(s), dishware and appliances for the kitchen, towels for the bathroom(s), and a sofa, table, television, and *farsh* (floor mattresses stuffed with sheep wool) for the *manzūl* (living/reception room). In 2007, I noticed that none of the summer weddings involved couples that were moving in with the groom's family. The couples were older (in their early twenties), as they had postponed getting married until they were able to secure the income to purchase land on which to build and furnish a house. The bridegroom who can furnish a house appears to be increasingly favored by women and their families. Reproducing families increasingly requires establishing a permanent independent household, which presupposes a viable occupation and income. In the context of Bedouin marriage and family formation in the twenty-first century, the new rule seems to be: no house, no marriage. For most Bedouins, the primary concern is not the prospect of losing their property (Bedouins are already land-poor), but the prospect of homelessness. Most Bedouins only "own" the small plot of land on which their house sits.

Continuing attention is needed to the social and economic conditions under which marriage and kinship are congealed and sustained. Different modes of production produce variable kinship and marriage structures. The structure of social space within a given mode of production must also be examined, as it mirrors and structures the division of labor. The spatiality of daily life is central to the reproduction of society.[38] Traditionally, Bedouin migrated and camped with close paternal kin, usually their father's brother(s). The basic segment of the tribe is the *bayt* (minimal lineage). It is the smallest political unit, which—together with other structurally similar units—forms the internal organization of the *fakhad* (maximal lineage). The *bayt* also constitutes the patrilineal descent group, which once comprised a residential camping unit for part, if not all, of the pastoral cycle. Bedouin families today live in permanent villages, not mobile camps. Almost all villages consist of members of the same tribe. Indeed, as previously mentioned, the land on which Bedouin homes and villages rest today were originally purchased and founded by brothers or members of the same minimal lineage.

It is possible that as villages grow in size, those who live in larger, less isolated or dispersed villages will be less likely to marry kin as they have increasing opportunities to meet alternative mates. Bedouin village communities are not isolated or closed systems but are characterized by boundary permeability.[39] Communities lose members as people die, marry out, emigrate, and establish residency in different regions or countries. Bedouin communities also add new members, especially through marriage and reproduction. Today, even though the Bedouin fertility rate has started to decline, population will continue to grow for some time, due to population momentum (built-in growth due to youthful age structures). Even in smaller dispersed populations, not everyone can marry their first cousin.

There are simply not enough cousins to go around, and, oftentimes, the age gap between cousins is so great as to make the match impractical.

And, not to be forgotten, parents and children (particularly those in wage-labor families) frequently subvert social rules in practice. Women and men of marriageable age may reject their family's interventions altogether and decide to elope instead. A young woman's heartrending suicide over an impending forced marriage induced several women of her generation to elope and paved the way for other Bedouin women to successfully negotiate their own marriages with familial support. In commenting on the bride-to-be's taking of her own life, the daughter of the late woman's close friend (whose own mother eloped shortly after her friend's suicide) explains: "*Rabbat ajyāl.* (She taught or molded generations.) Families in our village stopped [the practice of forced marriage] after that." Social actors negotiate, manipulate, and contest the normative order and often do so in ways that bespeak their conflicting socioeconomic and emotional interests. Through their micro-level marriage actions, individuals are not only responding to macro-level social forces; they are contributing to their shape and trajectory.

Conclusion

Kinship remains central to the configuration of marriage within Bedouin society. Marriage between the children of brothers and other agnates serves to both represent and reproduce kinship. However, nascent occupational diversification is beginning to modify kinship and marriage structures. Bedouin involved in wage work and rural trades have lower rates of consanguineous marriage than pastoralists and sharecroppers. Family cooperation (kin support) in labor is common to both pastoralism and sharecropping. Under wage labor, the family is no longer the economic unit of production. The individual is separated from the household and dependent on the market and the sale of labor power as a commodity in return for money. In short, the proletarianization of labor disrupts the family and weakens kinship structures, including kinship-based marriage. Closely tied to the growth of noncooperative or nonfamily work is the growth of commodity consumption, with its expanding link to romantic love. Greater participation in extrafamilial activities during childhood and adolescence, including attendance at school and worship at mosque, may serve to further change the context in which marriage and family formation take place. It remains to be seen whether such a changing confluence of factors—particularly the expansion of commodity relations (proletarianization) and socialization by nonfamily agents, as well as shrinking family sizes—will lead to a weakening of family ties and subsequent decline in Bedouin consanguineous unions or to a change in the meaning, if not the practice, of close-kin marriages.

In spite of occupational distinctions in the frequency of consanguineous marriage, most Bedouins acknowledge a broader kinship relation to their marriage partners. While a substantial minority of Bedouin women (born between the end of the French Mandate and 1985) married their first cousins, the vast majority of Bedouins (89 percent) from all occupational backgrounds, including wage laborers, married someone from the same tribe. The tribal ties of kinship crosscut occupational designations. The broader pattern of lineage endogamy irrespective of local modes of production suggests the actualization of a kinship-based social order. The next chapters take a closer look at the demographic gap between social strata by placing Bedouin demographic events in comparative political-economic context. As chapters 7 and 8 will show, the extent to which socioeconomic inequality engenders demographic inequality varies across time and space. Chapter 6 offers alternative ways of conceptualizing high fertility and its relationship to poverty, social inequality, and ill health.

6

Population and Poverty

A Capitalist Trap?

Global fertility decline has brought with it an idealization of the Western bourgeois family type,[1] or what has been dubbed as "the early stopping, gender-balanced, child-centered nuclear family."[2] While the large family is seen as a throwback to an era marked by high death rates and poverty, the small family is heralded as a modern historical watershed. The decline of mortality and fertility across various parts of the globe over the last century and a half is widely regarded as one of the most important social transformations in human history. This process, referred to as the demographic transition, is believed to consist of three major phases: pretransition (a historical period of equilibrium marked by high mortality and high fertility), transition (a period of destabilization in mortality and fertility rates as mortality declines and fertility remains high), and post-transition (a period of near equilibrium in which fertility declines, initiating a low-mortality and low-fertility regime).

The first wave of modern demographic transitions (as well as industrialization and urbanization) began in Europe and some parts of North America in the early eighteenth century.[3] In most of Europe, mortality began to decline in 1800,[4] and the fertility transition largely occurred between 1870 and 1960.[5] Between World War II and the early 1960s, there appeared to be stability on the world demographic scene, with sharp and wide divisions between rich and poor countries.[6] An important shift in the theoretical language used to describe the widening demographic distinctions between rich and poor countries also began at this time. As early as the eighteenth century, the interests of poor colonized people were not given much weight, except as subject peoples who needed to be brought to the same level of "civilization" as "superior" and more "evolved" Europeans. The responsibility for "civilizing," "educating" and subduing "backward" natives the world over was glossed as "white man's burden"—an idea premised on European racial superiority and power.[7]

After World War II, colonial language and institutions were modified somewhat. Foreign "aid" was ushered in with Harry Truman's Point Four Program. The terms "developed" and "underdeveloped" replaced "civilized" and "uncivilized," respectively. The phrase "the Third World"—coined by French demographer Alfred Sauvy in the wake of the cold war—drew attention to the struggle of capitalist countries in the West to control newly independent countries in the global South. A cold-war binary coexisted with Sauvy's tripartite scheme: the capitalist West, the communist bloc, and the Third World. The newly designated phrase "the Third World" was substituted for "savage peoples."[8] Today, the United Nations, one of the many agencies created in the aftermath of World War II, employs a similar classification scheme, distinguishing between "more developed," "less developed," and "least developed" countries. Not surprisingly, it is the "less" and "least developed" countries today that conform least to demographic transition theory's projections of mortality reductions. Several countries have experienced a reversal in life-expectancy gains predicted by the demographic-transition model. In sub-Saharan Africa, mortality actually rose in the 1990s due to HIV/AIDS, which has become the main cause of death. Countries in Eastern Europe and former territories of the Soviet Union have also experienced a decline in life expectancy over the past three decades, even prior to undergoing the arduous transition to a market economy.[9]

The classic demographic-transition model predicts that a decline in the death rate precedes a drop in the birth rate. Although the timing and pace of fertility decline varies considerably across countries and regions, there were clear-cut divisions between rich and poor countries in the 1960s. The total-period fertility rate (TPFR) of "more developed" countries was 2.7, while that of "less developed" countries was 6.0. Most variation was along a Northern-Southern Hemisphere trajectory. Japan and parts of Central, Eastern, and Northern Europe had a TPFR of less than 2.5. Only a few Southern Hemisphere countries of European descent (Argentina, Australia, New Zealand, and Uruguay) had moderately high fertility, with TPFRs from 2.5 to 4. However, the large majority of countries in Latin America, Africa, and Asia maintained very high levels of fertility (above 6.5).[10] The first wave of demographic transition was gradual and involved a few hundred million people.

By 1990–95, about three decades later, a dramatic change had occurred—fertility transition became a global phenomenon. The second wave of demographic transition—which included countries in the global South—was already in full swing. Mortality declined dramatically and with great rapidity in most regions, achieving in one or two decades what rich countries accomplished in one or two centuries. Fertility declines have occurred rapidly in East and Southeast Asia as well as Latin America, and more slowly in Africa.[11] Low-fertility countries (TPFRs below 2.5) now included Russia, all of Europe, Northern America, Australia, New Zealand, China, Thailand, and Brazil.[12] The decline of fertility over the last half century has been nothing short of striking. Between 1950–1955 and 2007, the fertility rate dropped across world regions of Africa (from 6.7 to 5.0), Asia (from 5.9 to 2.4), Latin America/Caribbean (from 5.9 to 2.5), North America (from 3.5 to 2.0), and Europe (from 2.7 to 1.5). As of 2007, only two regions remain with fertility rates above 5.5: sub-Saharan Africa (excluding Southern Africa) and Middle Eastern countries such as Yemen[13] and the 1967 occupied Palestinian territories.[14] However, even in Africa, countries with high total fertility rates (above 6.5) are largely limited to the Sahel zone and politically unstable areas.[15]

While the demographic gap has narrowed substantially, world demographic estimates for 2007 indicate that, on average, individuals in rich countries still have fewer children and live longer than those from poor countries. The average total fertility rate for the "more developed" countries is 1.6, and for the "less developed" countries is 2.9 if China is included, and 3.3 if China is excluded. The average life expectancy at birth for the "more developed" countries is 77 years, and for the "less developed" countries is 66 years if China is included, and 64 years if China is excluded.[16] Hence, while both the mortality and fertility gaps have closed over the past fifty years, the gap in fertility has closed more. In contrast, the economic gap (measured by per capita GDP) between high-income and low-income countries has widened during the past five decades.[17]

Some may believe that because mortality rates have fallen and fertility decline is now global, concerns about demographic polarization are now obsolete. However, this view obscures the fact that large shifts in age distributions and population sizes between regions and countries will continue over the next several decades. Demographers Paul Demeny and Geoffrey McNicoll point out that 99 percent of global population growth is expected to occur in the "less developed" regions, with approximately eighty million people being added every year, compared with about 1.6 million people in "more developed" countries. Whereas the "less developed" countries will keep growing (largely due to population momentum), causing an increase in the child dependency ratio (defined as the population aged zero to fourteen divided by the population aged fifteen to sixty-four), the "more developed" countries may grow slowly or not at all, leading to an increase in the old-age dependency ratio (defined as the number of those sixty-five and older divided by the population aged fifteen to sixty-four).[18] A major challenge for anthropological demographic theorizing is to understand the causes and consequences of demographic divides within and between countries. Explaining high and falling fertilities in their global, national, and local varieties is part of that task.

One of the main causes of high fertility is high mortality. Italian demographer Massimo Livi-Bacci proclaims that the reason population grew so slowly during the first 99 percent of human history was that death rates were very high, and the risk of death was particularly high among infants and young children.[19] Thus, people were forced to have a large number of children if they wanted to have even two or three survive to adulthood. Premodern life expectancies were believed to range from twenty to forty years[20] (compared to seventy-eight in the United States today), and under such conditions, women had to bear an average of more than four children each just to ensure that two would survive to adulthood. In those areas where mortality was even higher (such as India, where, as recently as 1900, life expectancy was less than twenty-seven years), women had to bear more than six children on average just to ensure that two would live to adulthood. In addition to behavioral replacement, there is a biological mechanism that links fertility and mortality. Deaths of nursing infants and young children in the first few years of life shorten the length of a birth interval, because such deaths terminate lactation, with its contraceptive effect. As a result, the mother is potentially exposed to pregnancy and birth sooner than she otherwise would have been.

The notion of a demographic equilibrium, whereby population grows slowly if at all because of high mortality, is itself a legacy of Malthusian theory. Political economist and father of demography Reverend Dr. Thomas Robert Malthus observed that, under the most favorable circumstances, human populations (like other biological populations) have the potential to increase geometrically or double every twenty-five years.[21] Assuming geometric or exponential growth, and that the population of the entire earth were one billion, and doubles every twenty-five years, then in one century the population would grow to 16 billion, in two centuries the population would grow to 256 billion, and in three centuries to 4,096 billion, and so on. However, such rapid population growth has not occurred. Malthus postulated that because population increases geometrically (due to what he believed to be the invariant biological urge to reproduce) and the food supply only increases arithmetically, there is an inevitable tension between population growth and the means of subsistence. The demographic imbalance or excess population is ultimately brought back in line with the level of subsistence by natural forces—the infamous Malthusian trap. That is, the population is checked by "the desolations of war, pestilence, famine and the convulsions of nature," or what Malthus referred to as positive checks to population.[22]

Malthus's "natural law of population" was an attempt to explain how the world was kept from being overrun by people. Positive checks on mortality meant that deaths exceeded births. However, Malthus also recognized the existence of "preventive checks" to population, which he believed were unique to humans. Preventive checks were largely voluntary and consisted of restraints on birth. The principal form of restraint enumerated and endorsed by Malthus was moral or prudential restraint from marriage. Malthus argued that in Europe, moral restraint was one of the most powerful checks to population—at least among the upper classes—that kept population down to the level of the means of subsistence.[23]

Critics have observed that because Malthus's positive checks really only apply to the poor, his proposed law is neither natural nor universal but can actually be broken down into class-specific laws—one for the rich and one for the poor.[24] The Malthusian model does suggest that the poor and "savage nations," including not only China and India but "the countries possessed by the Bedoween Arabs," were more vulnerable to positive checks and natural calamities.[25] Malthus does not attribute excessive reproduction to unjust structures of society or the lack of effective technological buffers against environmental stress and disease, but attributes it to immoral behavior—the alleged individual proclivity for vice (e.g., sex and alcohol in the case of England's poor). In other words, the Malthusian view proclaims that the lower classes are condemned to a life of misery governed by positive checks because they lack moral restraint, choosing to marry early and have large families regardless of their economic circumstances. Malthus believed that poverty, misery, and death were natural consequences of increasing too fast:

> Natural and moral evil seem to be the instruments employed by the Deity in admonishing us to avoid any mode of conduct which is not suited to our being, and will consequently injure our happiness. If we be intemperate in eating and drinking, we are disordered ... if we multiply too fast, we die miserably of poverty and contagious diseases.[26]

Not only is death a consequence of prolific reproduction, but Malthus's natural law envisions these "checks" as divine punishment for irrational and immoral behavior. The positive and preventive checks, as stipulated by Malthus, were class-specific in their conceptualization, with positive checks affecting the impoverished classes, not the rich. The rich supposedly warded off positive checks by postponing marriage and childbearing and practicing sexual restraint in the interim. As a result, the rich were believed to enjoy greater economic and social prosperity.

While Malthus recognized class differences, he tried to both naturalize and individualize them. Class is invoked only to be concealed. Hence, all we are left with is individual vice. The poor are poor because they are oversexed and lazy. The locus of responsibility is the individual. The inability to control one's urge to reproduce is the source of all misery. Accordingly, the solution to overpopulation is to effect a change in individual-level behavior, which Malthus believed had to be largely punitive—gradually abolish the poor laws. Human procreative behavior must be shaped through naked power and education.

Malthus enjoined England's laboring poor to depend upon their "own prudence and industry,"[27] particularly, prudence in the affair of marriage, and not rely on parish support. Malthus writes:

> The labouring poor, to use a vulgar expression, seems always to live from hand to mouth. Their present wants employ their whole attention; and they seldom think of the future. Even when they have an opportunity of saving, they seldom exercise it; but all that they earn beyond their present necessities goes, generally speaking to the alehouse. The poor laws may, therefore, be said both to diminish both the power and the will to save among the common people, and thus to weaken one of the strongest incentives to sobriety and industry, and consequently to happiness.[28]

Malthus recognized the existence of economic inducements behind marriage and procreation. He argued that the poor laws ought to be abolished because they remove the economic constraints behind reproduction. The behavior of the poor could be modified through coercion, negative inducements, or harsh economic disincentives. In effect, the poor needed to be disciplined and punished to effect a change in their behavior. Malthus argued that if the poor laws remained in place, then the nation's wealth would be squandered and industriousness among the poor would be undermined, as the laboring classes would lose the incentive to work and economic productivity would concomitantly decline. The poor laws would not only delay what he believed to be inevitable—positive checks—but would exacerbate those checks, leading to heightened poverty, famine, and "wretchedness."[29] Such a doom-and-gloom scenario leaves little question as to why demography, like economics, has earned the moniker "the dismal science." By individualizing the causes of poverty, Malthus's arguments served to veil structural inequalities and power dynamics. His arguments undermined collective action, social responsibility, and "institutional thinking." Prominent German intellectuals Karl Marx (1818–1883) and Friedrich Engels (1820–1895) recognized the political implications of Malthus's argument. Marx saw in Malthusian theory a pseudoscientific doctrine that exalts the ruling classes and condemns the poor "to live in celibacy and to die of hunger." Similarly, Engels rejected Malthus's law as an "open declaration of war of the bourgeoisie upon the proletariat."[30]

It is important to recognize that Malthus's law did not attribute high fertility to high mortality, but just the reverse. Death was the result of uncontrolled reproduction. Because individuals were prolific in their reproduction, Malthus reasoned, they suffered the consequences—high mortality induced by famine, disease, warfare, and so forth. Malthus understood that extreme poverty would in turn check population,[31] but it was high fertility due to individual flaws—imprudence and lack of sobriety—that was ultimately held responsible for creating a high-mortality regime. I do not wish to undermine key contributions of Malthusian theory. Today we recognize that the fertility-mortality link works both ways, as high fertility can also cause high mortality. When women have pregnancies too close together, this can increase the risk of death for young children.[32] Sociological demographers James Lee and Wang Feng credit Malthus for his recognition of different kinds of positive checks operant in human societies. Malthus distinguished between two varieties of positive checks—"volitional vice" and "involuntary constraint."[33] Volitional vice is regarded as a useful concept,[34] as it allows for discussion of endogenous, human-induced causes of mortality, such as infanticide or war.

However, other aspects of Malthusian theory need to be rejected, and yet others revised. Attempts to naturalize and individualize the causes of poverty without serious attention to structural inequalities should be rejected. In addition, Malthus's emphasis on positive checks as the primary force operating in human history to keep population in check warrants revision. We now know that different populations, both contemporary and historical, have been able to evade the Malthusian trap. Historical demographic research suggests that preventive checks have in many cases played an equal if not greater role in preventing population growth in human history.

For example, in their research on Chinese historical demography (using Chinese genealogies), Lee and Feng discovered that the Chinese demographic system was historically characterized by a low frequency of famines. Its population was kept in check by sociocultural practices like infanticide, used consciously by the Chinese to regulate both the size and the gender configuration of their families. The Chinese population was also kept in check by moderate levels of fertility achieved by delayed starting, early stopping, and long spacing. Long birth intervals were in large measure attributable to the Chinese practice of marital restraint, or the control of sexual activity within marriage. Marital restraint is part of a longer tradition of carnal restraint espoused by all major Chinese philosophies and religions, including Daoism, Confucianism, and Buddhism.[35] Hence, contra Malthus, the authors affirm the central importance of preventive checks in China's demographic history. It was only when these checks were destabilized during periods of political-economic and ecological upheaval that China experienced a population boom.[36] China is not unique in this regard, as historical demographic evidence from Japan,[37] precolonial Southeast Asia,[38] precolonial India,[39] and Indonesia[40] reveals that similar kinds of preventive checks and self-imposed positive checks served to limit population growth. Classism and racism prevented Malthus from seeing that preventive checks played an equally important role outside of an aristocratic European milieu.

Bedouin Health, Fertility and Economic Well-Being in Perspective

It is difficult for scholars and the general public to accept that high fertility can be achieved without negative socioeconomic and health consequences. Very high fertility in Bedouin communities did not occur at a time-space juncture marked by economic destitution or pauperism. Measures of socioeconomic well-being are relative. The average income and living standards of the Bekaa Valley's rural inhabitants fall below those of Beirut's residents. Within the Bekaa, there is clear evidence of socioeconomic and demographic distinctions between Bedouin and peasant groups. Most Bedouin do not own farmland and do not have home ownership and tenure security. Indeed their very status as Lebanese citizens is in question, which puts them at a serious disadvantage when trying to access government-related services and opportunities in education, health, and employment. Poverty is a relative and multidimensional concept, but my focus here is on the nutritional health implications of poverty. People suffering from undernutrition are generally poor, but not all poor people are undernourished.[41]

Anthropometry is the most useful method for assessing the nutritional health status of individuals and population groups. Weight-for-height, or body mass index (BMI), is now widely regarded as the most objective anthropometric indicator of nutritional status in adults. Bedouin women's

BMI status shows that they have sufficient energy stores within the body and thus overall nutritional and dietary adequacy. For most people, BMI correlates with their amount of body fat. The mean BMI for Bedouin women ages fifteen to fifty-four in 2000 is 26.7 kg/m² (SD = 5.7). The BMI of their spouses who were present at the time of the interviews was also calculated and yielded a mean value of 27.3 kg/m² (SD = 5.6), but this should be considered a tentative BMI estimate at best, as the sample size was very small (N = 17). BMI for women varies significantly with age, but not by occupation or wealth. The mean BMI values broken down by age are 25.7 kg/m² (SD = 4.9) for younger women (15–39) and 29.7 kg/m² (SD = 6.8) for older women (forty and over) in 2000. According to the Centers for Disease Control and Prevention, an adult BMI of 18.5 constitutes the minimum threshold for health and fitness. A BMI below 18.5 is considered a low weight for height and carries an increased risk of health problems. A BMI between 18.5 and 24.9 is considered a healthy weight for adults.[42] A BMI between 25.0 to 29.9 is considered overweight and a BMI of 30 or higher is considered obese. Both younger and older Bekaa Bedouin women are in the overweight range. Declining activity levels and the dietary changes that have accompanied the Bedouin transition to a sedentary lifestyle are probably responsible for the high BMI (weight/height) status of women. Being overweight makes women more vulnerable to cardiovascular disease and diabetes mellitus. Bedouins are a rapidly modernizing population undergoing profound changes in terms of life expectancy, nutrition, and patterns of disease—the so-called "epidemiological transition." One of the consequences of higher modern life expectancy due in part to improved nutrition is that the chronic diseases of old age have increasingly replaced parasitic and degenerative diseases.

The Bekaa Bedouin case illustrates the conditions under which people can have high fertility without falling into the Malthusian trap of high death rates spurred by disease, food insecurity, and undernutrition. As chapter 3 reveals, very high fertility (TFR = 9.08) among the Bekaa Bedouin is found in conjunction with moderate levels of infant mortality (0.05), moderate child mortality (0.01), and minor gender differences in health. Bedouin health falls below that of their peasant neighbors in Lebanon, but when compared to the global average, or to other nomadic groups around the world (see chapter 8 for a comparative discussion of infant and child health in nomadic communities), Bedouin fare pretty well. Estimates of life expectancy, another common measure of population health, shows that Bedouins can expect to live relatively long lives. Bedouin life expectancy is about sixty-five years—a figure that falls between the global average life expectancy in 2000, estimated at sixty-six years, and the average life expectancy for "less developed" countries in 2000, estimated at sixty-four years.

One of the main reasons why high Bedouin fertility (four times higher than the national TFR for Lebanon) did not lead to impoverishment is because of the low consumption levels in their society. This allowed Bedouin families to escape the Malthusian trap. Childbearing and child-rearing did not entail great expense prior to and at the early onset of sedentarization. The costs associated with Bedouin household and family formation (e.g., getting married, building and furnishing a house, child educational expenses, etc.) were low. Up until the 1960s, Bedouin relied on camels for transport and few had permanent households. Children did not attend school and began to contribute to the household economy by the age of eleven or so. Bedouin were not burdened with expenses that plagued their settled peasant neighbors—they did not have electricity and consequently lacked expenses associated with modern appliances (washing machine, refrigerator, television, stereo, lighting, gas stoves to replace traditional wood-burning or kerosene stoves, etc.); they did not have educational expenses (school fees, books/supplies) or hired labor (Bedouins relied on family labor); and they did not purchase store-bought clothing, makeup, and expensive food.

It was not until the 1970s and 1980s that Bedouins began settling down and constructing permanent households. Absent consumer outlays associated with sedentarization, it was possible to have many children without living in poverty. The Bedouin can be characterized as a low-consumption society marked by hard work and collective family labor. It is the same feature shared by other community-oriented classless societies such as the Anabaptist Hutterites and the Old Order Amish in North America. The latter groups enjoyed higher fertility than the national U.S. average without experiencing a Malthusian disaster. Old Order Amish prosperity can, in large part, be attributed to simpler farming methods—requiring essentially only a horse-drawn plow or, in the case of a dairy farm, simple hand-milking techniques—and reliance on the work contribution of the entire family (no hired labor) as well as the imperatives of self-abnegation and restrained consumption.[43] As a result, Anabaptist groups, much like the Bekaa Bedouin, were able to maintain high fertility without facing negative social or health consequences. Thus, it is problematic to argue that in contemporary very-high-fertility groups, high fertility is invariably the result of high mortality. Empirical evidence suggests that very high fertility and low mortality characterize both Bedouins and Hutterites.[44] Perhaps above all this is because Bedouins and Hutterites have some access to modern health-care facilities, skilled midwifery, and high-quality weaning foods in the form of domesticated animal milk. Taken together, we can say that very high Bedouin fertility, moderate mortality and high BMI are an instantiation of adequate food and nutrition—perhaps even overnutrition,[45] not infectious disease, early death, and pauperism.

A historically situated perspective of high Bedouin fertility shows that high fertility extends back to the French colonial period in Syria and Lebanon and continues post-independence—a period of rapid urbanization and rural industrialization in the region.[46] At the proximate level, high Bedouin fertility was achieved through a long reproductive span, short interbirth intervals (due to early weaning), low rates of sterility, and high rates of marital stability. A fundamental sociodemographic shift occurred in the 1960s, with the replacement of camels with pickup trucks, which greatly reduced the mobility of Bedouin pastoralists. Just as camels were sold to purchase pickup trucks, sheep and goats were sold (either all or part of the herd) to purchase land and build a house. Villagization and rural industrialization precipitated a decline in Bedouin pastoralism and an increase in agricultural sharecropping and wage labor. Once Bedouins lost access to the means of production (in terms of livestock and grazing lands), they became increasingly reliant on their labor for survival. Indeed, the historical increase in Bedouin fertility (i.e., women born between 1934 and 1960) appears to be linked to the increasing demand for labor occasioned by the economic shift from nomadic pastoralism to agricultural sharecropping and wage labor. However, this process did not necessarily involve conscious decision-making. While there is some evidence among the Bedouin of conscious control of fertility within marriage—achieved by willfully suspending social practices that regulate births (i.e., breastfeeding and coitus interruptus)—most hard-worked Bedouin women probably had less time for on-demand feeding and, consequently, experienced repeated interruption of breastfeeding due to pregnancy. A positive feedback loop is likely to have occurred with increased labor inputs into agriculture inadvertently causing high fertility, which necessitated labor intensification to meet the growing subsistence needs of the family, which, in turn, led to further reductions in breastfeeding and higher fertility.[47]

Over the long term, however, the Bedouin economic transition from pastoralist to (landless) peasant and from pastoralist to proletariat drove Bedouin fertility downward. Settled Bedouin communities confronted a different social and economic order, one that increasingly involved weighing expenses and coming to terms with growing demands on the household exchequer. In terms of fertility behavior, Bedouin families have adjusted to these new constraints in their sociocultural environment by controlling their fertility within marriage. A drop in Bedouin fertility can be seen among women born after 1970 and who began their childbearing in the late 1980s and early 1990s. The total-period fertility rate (TPFR) at the time of the demographic interviews in 2000 was 6.55—an almost 30 percent drop from the total-cohort fertility rate (TCFR) found among older postreproductive women. Newly wedded couples interviewed in 2007 during the peak-summer marriage season, indicated a desire for two to three children on average. When explaining their small desired family size, young brides explained that they wanted to be able to provide a good education for their children and feed them well. They also emphasized the importance of sending their children to school dressed appropriately—wearing decent shoes and clothes and having the necessary school supplies. As the costs of children were raised by changes in the sociopolitical and economic landscape, and as consumer aspirations rose, fertility declined. The economic challenges facing Bedouins undergoing villagization, particularly those related to household and family formation altered the consumption-population nexus. Once the consumption-population nexus changed, so too did fertility. The transition to low fertility among the Bedouin appears to be a transition to economic hardship in a new consumer society.

With increasing Bedouin integration into peasant village and town life, the costs of production and reproduction have increased dramatically. The mechanization of transport, privatization of land, and the commoditization of land and labor power have amplified Bedouin reliance on money. Bedouin pastoralists must pay to rent land in order to graze their flocks. Because migration to Syria is no longer part of the winter pastoral cycle, Bedouin pastoralists are more reliant on purchased feedstuffs (which include hay and sugar-beet pulp) and vitamins in the winter. Barns or pens now protect livestock from the winter cold, and purchased feed (as opposed to natural grasses) are increasingly used to sustain flocks. As one Bedouin man proclaimed: "It used to be that sheep and goats ate natural grasses. Today, they eat money." Such statements illustrate what Marx calls the transformation of a use-value into a commodity. Sharecropping households are also dependent on money as a medium of exchange. When entering into sharecropping agreements, Bedouin families need money to purchase seeds, fertilizers, and insecticides. In addition, trucks require maintenance, repair, and fuel expenses.

The historical decline of Bedouin pastoralism is cause for concern, since a mixed economy allows for diversification of income, which appears to provide a nutritional advantage. Recent studies of Bedouin children's food consumption and nutritional status in different parts of Lebanon revealed that nutritional deprivation was more pronounced among settled Bedouins who received rations from the government than Bedouins who had a diversified subsistence base. Bedouin children in the Bekaa were found to have better nutritional status than Bedouin children in other parts of Lebanon. The higher nutritional status of Bekaa Bedouin children was attributed to income derived from small-scale cash-crop production, livestock milk production, and wage labor.[48] Supplementary income derived from wage labor was afforded in large part by massive rural-to-urban migration on the part of peasants. Virtually all Bekaa Bedouin households, regardless of their dominant form of production, rely on the extra income derived from seasonal wage labor. Overreliance on wage labor is dangerous in the long term, as it makes peoples more vulnerable to cycles of accumulation and dispossession. Hence, a mixed agropastoral economy, based on access to the means of production, is central to understanding the demographic and nutritional profiles of the Bekaa Bedouin. As more and more Bedouin families relinquish their herds (to buy land or build a house) and lose a fundamental part of their economic livelihoods, a future decline in their overall health is likely to occur. Ownership of livestock provides a buffer against nutrition- and health-related impoverishment. Prospective research is necessary to determine whether or not greater integration of Bedouins into a global capitalist economy will result in poorer nutrition.

The costs associated with establishing an independent household have placed considerable strain on Bedouin families. Young couples need money to buy land and build a house. Whereas the oldest son and his bride can share residence with his family, constraints imposed by space and convention preclude accommodating additional married couples in the parental household. To make matters more difficult, the demand for costly home accoutrements has grown considerably. Couples wish to install hot water heaters, tile flooring, and cabinet hardware, as well as furnish their homes with couches, beds, dressers, tables, and so forth sold at local furniture galleries. Other desired houseware and hardware items include kitchen appliances, lighting, doors, china, eating utensils, towels, bedding, and linens. Bedouin cultural dress has also undergone important transformations. Unlike their mothers, who wore the traditional *'uṣba* (black Bedouin headscarf) and *thawb* (long dress), younger Bedouin women, like their peasant neighbors, prefer colorful headscarves with coordinated dress/skirt/pants and fashionable shoes. Makeup is also a growing part of younger women's consumer lifestyle. In contrast to older Bedouin mothers, who simply wear kohl and color their hair with henna, younger women's grooming habits increasingly include use of foreign and counterfeited cosmetic products. The heightened pace of modernity has ushered in a brave new world of consumption. While Bedouin consumption is low by U.S. consumption standards, it clearly impacts Bedouin household income, which averages between US$200 and $300 per month.

Commoditization and sedentarization have altered the social and political-economic context of child-rearing and family formation. In short, the costs of education, housing, furniture, clothing, transportation, inputs into agropastoral production, and the lost income of children with schooling have all precipitated a decline in Bedouin fertility. Rising inflation in the late 1980s made it even more difficult for Bedouin families to maintain a viable household. After four decades of exchange-rate stability (including years of civil strife and fighting), the Lebanese pound depreciated rapidly in the 1986–1987 period.[49] At the end of 1986, the General Labor Federation of Lebanon estimated that during the first ten months of 1986, the cost of living for a family of five had risen by 150 percent. Monthly expenditure on basic items—excluding education, rent, and medical expenses—had risen from L£5,652 to L£14,083. Overall, the federation estimated that 1986 had witnessed a 226 percent increase in prices. By March 1987, the federation reported a 250 percent inflation rate, with food prices having increased 300 percent over the previous twelve months.[50] The downward turn of the Lebanese economy in the 1980s helped induce Bedouin fertility decline. Bedouin couples beginning their childbearing in the twenty-first century express a clear desire to limit their family size, stemming from concerns over the economic costs of raising children and maintaining a viable household. As a result, many younger women are increasingly turning to modern contraception, particularly the IUD and the pill. However, traditional forms of contraception (i.e., withdrawal and breastfeeding) were the most common forms of contraception employed by older women for spacing or late stopping.

When examining the broader trajectory of Bedouin fertility, it is clear that the period of very high fertility was of limited historical duration and should be situated in the broader context of demographic transition. In other words, to understand how groups like the Bekaa Bedouin maintained high fertility in the context of low to moderate mortality prior to fertility transition, it is necessary to consider the temporal scale at which demographic levels are being examined. Demographic transition theory predicts that a decline in the birth rate follows the decline in the death rate after a time lag. The historical "lag time," as demographers call it, can last years and even decades. It is believed that it takes time for people to adjust to the fact that mortality is actually lower and effect a change in their procreative behavior. The Bedouin time lag appears to have lasted approximately thirty years.

In contrast, the Hutterites of the North American plains maintained very high fertility for sixty years.[51] What is more, both fertility transitions occurred after mortality decline and as a consequence of changes accompanying modernization and capitalist expansion. The decline in Bekaa Bedouin fertility appears to be linked to increasing economic hardship, evidenced in the growing proportion of Bedouin families employed in wage labor and the growing costs associated with sedentary life (see chapter 2). Similar historical processes appear to have occurred in Hutterite colonies of the United States. That is, capitalist developments in agriculture in the North American plains resulted in technological change, greater agricultural specialization, and increases in the price of land, which inhibited further expansion of many Hutterite colonies.[52] The Bedouin and Hutterites were able to maintain very high fertility without experiencing poverty, since their frugal communal living and hard agricultural labor shielded them from the economic checks imposed by capitalism. However, over the long term, their new economic circumstances prompted them to control their fertility within marriage. A principal error in Malthusian reasoning lies in attributing his law of surplus population with its accompanying positive checks to "nature" rather than to the historically specific workings of the capitalist mode of production. As Marx observes, the surplus population to which Malthus refers in his natural law is:

> a necessary product of accumulation or of the development of wealth on a capitalist basis, this surplus population becomes, conversely, the lever of capitalistic accumulation, nay, a condition of existence of the capitalist mode of production. It forms a disposable industrial reserve army, that belongs to capital quite as absolutely as if the latter had bred it at its own cost. . . . it creates, for the changing needs of the self-expansion of capital, a mass of human material always ready for exploitation.[53]

Marx maintained that different cycles of accumulation and phases of the industrial expansion and contraction were accompanied by corresponding changes in the demand for labor. It is the process of accumulation (the appropriation by capitalists of surplus value produced by the labor power s/he buys) that produces a relative surplus population and poverty, not some fixed sexual urge to reproduce. Rather than put forth an abstract universal law of population, Marx proposes that "every specific historic mode of production has its own special laws of population, historically valid within its limits alone."[54] For Marx and Engels, solving the problems of poverty and so-called overpopulation required abolishing capitalism (with its exploitative class relations) and replacing it with socialism.

Conclusion

We know that human population grew slowly for most of human history, with explosive growth occurring around 1850—the time of the Industrial Revolution. Although Malthus argues that the size of the population is determined by both positive and preventive checks, he emphasized the primacy of positive checks in keeping human population low. Classic demographic transition theory also envisions a pretransitional phase marked by a demographic equilibrium of high mortality and high fertility. However, recent historical evidence suggests that pretransitional societies were not uniformly characterized by high fertility and high mortality—what is referred to as a high-pressure demographic system. This implies that pretransitional stability can be achieved via preventive checks that limit reproduction. In short, Malthus underestimated the pervasiveness of preventive checks in human demographic history, particularly among nonelite groups in Europe and beyond. Births can be kept in check by a variety of mechanisms, including moral restraint, marital restraint, breastfeeding spacing, abortion, and infanticide. The Bedouin case further illustrates that high mortality and poverty-induced famine are not inevitable consequences of high fertility. Very high Bedouin fertility—linked to rural industrialization and increasing reliance on agriculture—was of limited historical duration, "lagging behind" mortality for about thirty years. During that time, Bedouin were able to avert a Malthusian catastrophe, owing in large part to their internal egalitarian social structure and its attendant features of communal sharing, frugality, solidarity, and hard work. Anabaptist communities in North America were similarly successful in circumventing poverty and ill health in spite of their high fertility.

7

Class Differentiation of Demographic Regimes

It is generally acknowledged that one of the most important contributions to the anthropological and sociological study of demography over the last twenty-five years or so has been the identification of class/caste and occupational differentials in fertility and mortality within local communities at different stages of demographic transitions. Evidence of social-class variation in microfertility behavior has helped to rewrite our understanding of human demography, as it directly challenged the prevailing view among demographers that cultural/ideational, rather than material/economic, forces drive demographic change. My aim here is to examine these (mostly rural) empirical case studies and their implications for understanding class-related demographic differentiation across time-space. In doing so, I hope to identify some of the demographic and social mechanisms that lie behind class inequalities (or the lack thereof) in peasant communities, which can reciprocally inform our reading of class differentiation in nomadic communities discussed in the following chapter.

The results from the Princeton European Fertility Project constitute the main source of support for ideational arguments. The European Fertility Project is regarded as being one of the most important and ambitious undertakings in the social sciences to understand the demographic histories of Europe. In 1963, under the supervision of Ansley Coale at Princeton, researchers utilized relatively detailed quantitative data available for the several hundred administrative subdivisions of the nation-states of Europe to document and explain the historical decline in fertility, which had taken place between 1870 and 1960. In addition to putting out eleven volumes over a twenty-year period, the European Fertility Project published a summary volume in 1986, which basically concluded that socioeconomic factors (e.g., degree of urbanization, levels of education, and mortality) are less important than cultural factors (see below) for understanding the timing and patterning of fertility decline in European countries. In particular, language, religion, and customs or values were found to be the most important determinants of the onset of fertility transitions within national population.[1]

For example, in examining the history of fertility decline in Belgium, Ron Lesthaeghe found that linguistic factors account for much of the variation in the decline of marital fertility. Lesthaeghe determined that French-speaking areas of the country experienced fertility decline much earlier (often by several decades) than Flemish-speaking ones, even though the communities being compared had similar socioeconomic characteristics and were located in close geographical proximity.[2] While Lesthaeghe found differences in fertility behavior according to linguistic composition of districts, Livi-Bacci finds that religious and regional factors best explain family limitation patterns in Portugal. The onset of fertility decline in Portugal occurred first in the south of the country, even though the north was more industrialized. Livi-Bacci points to religious differences between a Catholic north and Protestant south in order to explain the differential timing of Portuguese marital fertility decline.[3] In an attempt to explain these and other similar findings, Susan Watkins proposed that culturally similar areas (in terms of language, religion, ethnic background, and lifestyle) were more likely to share a decline in fertility than areas that were culturally less similar. Watkins attributes the uniform demographic experiences of distinct cultural groups to the existence of shared communication communities (afforded by language), which allow ideas of family planning to diffuse quickly until they reach a cultural or geographic barrier to their further spread. As a result, once ideas of family limitation took root, they spread very quickly within provinces and nations that shared a common culture.[4]

Similarly, in reviewing the European Fertility Project's findings on historical Europe and data on the developing world (obtained from forty-one developing countries collected for the World Fertility Survey), John Cleland and Christopher Wilson conclude that it is the "culture" of subpopulations, loosely defined by religion, language, or region, that exerts primary influence on the patterning of reproductive change. The authors contend that peoples within cultural groups or regions tend to be relatively homogeneous in their fertility-decline experiences, in spite of the fact that regions often exhibit considerable internal variation in levels of socioeconomic development, education, or in the availability of family-planning services.[5] Cleland and Wilson uphold the primacy of broader social forces in explaining marital fertility decline in Europe:

The fact that, within culturally homogeneous populations, birth control and resulting marital fertility decline spreads to all sectors within a remarkably short period of time implies that the fundamental forces of change operated at the societal level. The household economics model seems an entirely inappropriate framework for understanding a change of this nature, because of the vast differences in micro-economic realities of households in transitional societies. The explanation must surely be sought in changes that can be experienced in common. This does not preclude broad economic factors, but strongly suggests the influence of new knowledge, ideas, and aspirations that can spread independently of individual economic circumstances.[6]

While fertility differentials within geographically and culturally defined units were deemed minor or negligible, cultural differences between groups were deemed to be of primary importance for understanding fertility decline. In other words, when it comes to the fertility transition, there was believed to be cultural homogeneity within, but cultural difference without. While the authors do not rule out the importance of broader economic factors (e.g., the spread of industrial capitalism, urbanization, and nationalism), in understanding demographic transition in Europe over the course of the nineteenth and twentieth centuries, they conclude that noneconomic factors best account for the timing and spread of transitions within Europe.

The emphasis on cultural factors for understanding European fertility decline was a major impetus that drove demography closer to anthropology and anthropological methods of inquiry.[7] Anthropologists, however, tend to be critical of large-scale demographic studies, because such highly aggregated analyses are believed to mask variation in local-level behavior. In order to address the question as to what determines family size and what causes people to alter their fertility behavior via starting, spacing or stopping, critics reason, attention should be shifted from the macro societal level to the micro individual level. Local cases studies allow researchers to better understand how people actually respond, in terms of their reproductive behavior, to constraints and opportunities in their sociocultural and biophysical environments. Such has been the focus of microdemographic studies in sociocultural anthropology and related social-science disciplines. While some anthropologists have called for an entirely new kind of demographic analysis: a "demography without numbers,"[8] others have argued for a "thicker demography"[9] or "whole demographies"[10]—studies that combine qualitative and quantitative approaches[11] as well as ethnographic and demographic approaches.[12] In contrast to macrodemographic research, microdemographic studies tend to emphasize reproductive heterogeneity, not homogeneity, and tend to highlight the importance of socioeconomic factors, particularly class, for understanding demographic variation and change at the local level.

The Role of Class in Microdemographic Explanation

Several microdemographic studies have documented social variation in demographic behavior in general and social class/caste or occupational differences in particular. Anthropological and sociological research in European societies has revealed the presence of class-specific demographic differentials at the local community level in Casalecchio, Italy,[13] and Villamaura (Sicily)[14] during the fertility transition. David Kertzer and Dennis Hogan, using parish register data in Italy, and Schneider and Schneider, using civil register data in Sicily, confirm that upper and middle classes in both local settings began family limitation sooner than other class groups. The fertility of the landed elites declined first, followed by that of artisans, merchants, and wage laborers later in the nineteenth and twentieth centuries. Directly prior to fertility decline, demographic differences among emergent classes were also discernable, although the direction of the relationship was reversed, with landowning elites having higher fertility than other groups.[15]

The work of Kertzer and Hogan as well as that of Schneider and Schneider has led to a refinement of the European Fertility Project's findings that whole regions undergo demographic transition simultaneously by revealing how three independent fertility transitions occurred within the same community. Their research helped demonstrate how different classes living in the same locality reduced their fertility at different times and in response to different political-economic and legal forces of change. For example, Kertzer and Hogan found that in the northern Italian town of Casalecchio, while the marital fertility of the elite class declined first, as was true for most of Europe, other social classes, such as wage laborers, continued to have large numbers of children until the costs of children were raised by changing political-economic conditions. Specifically, during the second half of the nineteenth century, the disappearance of service as an early life stage increased the costs of children in wage-earner families by extending their stay in the natal household.[16] Likewise, compulsory school-attendance laws and the passage of increasingly restrictive labor laws regulating children's factory work reduced the economic value of children, leading to family-size limitation among the proletariat. Sharecroppers also experienced an independent transition, continuing to have large families well into the twentieth century.[17] Again, their fertility only declined when the role of children in the family economy changed. The declining economic value of children was tied to the disappearance of sharecropping contracts with the increased capitalization of agriculture.[18]

Schneider and Schneider similarly attempt to explain the class specificity of demographic transition in Sicily, as well as the distinct political-economic changes that brought about each of the successive declines. In explaining the fertility transition among artisans, Schneider and Schneider argue that historical processes served to alter the practice of apprenticeship, which was crucial to artisans who expected their male children to follow their example, since "Shoemakers make shoemakers, [and] carpenters make carpenters."[19] However, since most child apprentices earned no income and required specialized training from craftsmen outside of their village in Palermo, apprenticeships entailed considerable expense. With the depression of the interwar years, currency devaluations, and restrictions on emigration to North America, apprenticeships became an even greater burden, particularly in the face of bleak employment prospects. As a result, artisans began to embrace the idea of "the small, early-stopping family" so that they could continue to provide children with respectable economic opportunities for their class in the face of economic hardship.[20] Artisan families were concerned with safeguarding a precious resource (i.e., skills) that a growing underclass did not possess.[21] Family limitation among Sicilian artisans was thus motivated by a desire to protect their livelihood, respected social position, and cultural identity.

The fertility transition of Sicily's *braccianti* class (landless laborers) in the 1950s and 1960s requires a slightly different interpretation. While Schneider and Schneider point to the rising cost of children in postwar Sicily in terms of birth and child care, education, clothing, and recreational activities, the primary inducement behind family limitation appeared to be opportunity, as opposed to constraint.[22] Most *braccianti* families began to use contraception after 1950 in order to seize upon the benefits of economic development and rising standards of living. Increased economic prosperity was ushered in, with external Marshall Plan aid from the United States and internal agrarian and industrial reforms in Italy. These political-economic developments not only paved the way toward national health, welfare, and pension plans but expanded the number of good-paying public-sector jobs for which Sicilians and south Italians could compete.[23] Hence, Schneider and Schneider emphasize that unlike the transition among gentry and artisan groups, who were motivated by a desire to protect their class standing, for most members of the *braccianti* class, the transition to low fertility was motivated by a desire to improve their socioeconomic status and acquire a more respectable life.[24]

Class differences in the onset and pace of fertility transition have also been found in rural England. Barry Reay's examination of three adjoining parishes in the Blean area of Kent reveals that prior to fertility transition (i.e., cohorts of women born between 1800 and 1834), farmers had the highest fertility, followed by the laboring and trades/crafts occupations.[25] It is clear that women marrying between 1835–49 and 1850–64 were reducing their family sizes in the Blean parishes, and the pace of fertility decline was quicker for farming families. During the marriage cohort of 1850–80, farming couples were marrying at a much later age than trades/crafts or laboring couples, largely in response to agricultural crisis as well as the introduction of the New Poor Law in 1834, and reduced their completed family size from 8.8 to 4.1.[26] Differences in infant and child mortality were not pronounced but indicate lower mortality for children of landowning farmers.[27]

Caste/Class Differentials in Non-European Societies

While the relationship between class and local demographic patterns outside of Europe is less understood, class/caste differences during transition have been found in Punjab, India,[28] and west-central Nepal.[29] In an examination of eleven villages in Ludhiana District, Punjab, Monica Das Gupta documents the presence of caste/class differentials in fertility in Punjab, India, among the Jat landowning caste and the Chamar caste of landless laborers. The Indian example parallels the European situation in that it is the upper classes that were the first to limit their family sizes. Das Gupta shows that fertility decline, which began around 1940, occurred earlier and more rapidly among landowners than among the landless.[30]

To explain the earlier timing and quicker pace of fertility decline in the landowning group, Das Gupta describes how landowners benefited from improvements in mortality sooner than landless families. Development efforts increased the predictability and magnitude of agricultural yields, which enhanced the sense of security and control that people had over their lives. Landed classes were also more mindful of status considerations, particularly that of keeping the family estate intact. Under customs or laws stipulating partible inheritance, improvements in child survival placed excess pressure on land resources, making intergenerational downward mobility increasingly likely for landowning families. Hence, in order to protect their class/

caste standing and ensure that the next generation would have sufficient land to support a family, landowning groups began to limit their fertility.[31] According to Das Gupta, large families did not pose the same threat to landless families, whose livelihood was only indirectly tied to land. Nevertheless, within a short span of time, the landless began to reduce their fertility in response to economic imperatives. In particular, as landowners abandoned their patron-client relationship to reduce labor expenses, the landless were left with a dwindling income base and increased economic pressure to reduce their fertility.[32]

In studying the fertility of caste-Hindus in Nepal who reside in an administrative unit composed of three villages, Steven Folmar similarly finds intrasocietal fertility variation immediately prior to and at the onset of fertility decline. Prior to fertility transition, the elite or large-farm high castes had the highest fertility, whereas small-farm high castes had the lowest fertility. The small-farm high castes and the low castes have recently begun to limit their fertility with modern contraception; however the fertility of elite large-farm high castes remains high and unrestricted.[33]

At first, it may seem surprising to note that small-farm high castes experienced fertility decline before large-farm high castes. Folmar explains that high castes with smaller land holdings faced more pressing economic constraints, which served to "check" their reproductive capacity to a greater extent than high castes with more sizable land holdings. In Nepal, marriage is often followed by a period of up to two years during which the bride lives in her father's home. However, this period tends to be longer among small-farm high castes, because they have fewer resources to support a new bride.[34] Likewise, high-caste women living on small farms tend to observe post-widowhood celibacy to a greater degree than women residing on large farms, since the economic resources of the latter allow them to absorb additional children, who frequently accompany remarriage, with greater ease.[35] Das Gupta similarly observes that those with larger land holdings in Punjab, India, did not restrict marriage to the same extent as those with smaller land holdings. The determining factor was land—when land was scarce or insufficient to support a family, subdivision became a concern and marriage restriction invoked.[36]

Taken together, case studies drawn from peasant societies in Europe, India, and Nepal provide empirical support for local demographic heterogeneity according to caste and class affiliation during demographic transitions. However, our understanding of the role of social class in shaping the demographic experiences of Western and non-Western peoples would not be complete without considering the demographic implications of class differences before fertility transition. A critical limitation of research on social-class variation in pretransitional societies is that most of literature is confined to Western Europe. Nevertheless, as Watkins suggests, it is imperative to examine demographic regimes prior to transition "because the characteristics of western European populations before transition influence their subsequent trajectories"[37] and also because reproductive homogeneity constitutes a sort of "confirmed generalization" for human populations prior to transition.

Local Class Differences in Pretransitional Western Europe

Most demographers believe that natural fertility patterns were uniform prior to the onset of an irreversible decline. The model fertility schedules compiled by Ansley Coale and James Trussell served to establish the age pattern of childbearing found across most human populations.[38] Hence, the assumption of local reproductive homogeneity is based on the almost universal finding from decades of demographic research on natural-fertility populations that female fertility exhibits a standard age pattern. That is, women experience a peak in their reproduction in their early twenties, after which point marital fertility begins to decline until it approaches zero in the late forties, forming a convex curve or pattern. The convex pattern of parity-independent fertility is well accepted. It is generally understood that the universal age pattern of fertility in natural-fertility populations is a function of both biological mechanisms (e.g., declining fecundity with age) and behavioral mechanisms (e.g., declining coital frequency), although biological factors affecting female fecundity are believed to be of primary importance.[39]

While age-related changes in reproductive function are universal, this does not mean that social variation between populations is absent. Nor does the concept of natural fertility preclude variation in fertility levels within the same population in different time periods. Indeed, levels of fertility may be very different between societies or within the same society at different points in time—reflected in differences in the height of fertility curves. Nevertheless, the similar shape of the curves suggests a common underlying pattern in the age structure of fertility. Exceptions to the convex pattern are found among unique subgroups of "social forerunners" within larger communities. Specifically, Livi-Bacci suggests that social differences in Europe prior to transition are largely confined to urban-rural differences with urban elites—ruling families, nobility, and bourgeoisie—pioneering family-limitation practices.[40]

Microdemographic studies showing fertility differentials within local communities are few, but they are not entirely lacking. For example, pronounced occupational differences in fertility were revealed in a dynamic analysis of a group of French parishes in the city of Rouen from 1700–1789.[41] Specifically, rich and poor segments of the population were shown to have different fertility responses to fluctuations in the price of wheat. The urban poor (laborers) experienced a dramatic drop in their fertility in response to price increases, whereas the fertility of the urban wealthy (notables and artisans) was virtually unaffected. Because Patrick Galloway found that fertility responses to price changes were independent of mortality effects, were the same for total births and legitimate births, and were not affected by migration or spousal separation, he concludes that voluntary marital fertility control was being practiced by the urban poor[42] during periods of economic hardship or crisis. Susan Scott and Christopher Duncan have uncovered modest fertility differentials among three social classes in the rural parish of Penrith in northern England for the years 1600–1800. The total marital fertility of elites (7.6) was higher than that of tradesmen (6.9) and subsistence (6.0) groups. It appears that, at the proximate level, intergroup differences were largely due to differences in birth-interval length, which were in turn linked to differences in breastfeeding practices.[43]

While few studies establish social-class variation in fertility prior to transition, social-class differentials in mortality have been confirmed in several European localities. In Rouen, Galloway found that poor segments of the urban population had higher infant mortality and lower life expectancy at birth during the second half of the eighteenth century. Life expectancy at birth for notables was 32.5 years and that of laborers 24.5—a difference of approximately eight years.[44] Other studies reveal that class differences in mortality prior to transition are not confined to urban populations. A rural study by Jona Schellekens on the mortality levels of different socioeconomic groups (farmers, cottagers, and laborers) in Gilze and Rijen, two eighteenth-century Dutch villages, shows that there were large differences in mortality between farmers and agricultural laborers. The estimated difference between the life expectancies of the lower and upper classes exceeds ten years.[45] Schellekens finds that malnutrition does not account for social disparities in mortality during the eighteenth century, since there was no significant correlation between the price of rye—the main cereal consumed—and child mortality among children of agricultural laborers. While mortality crises among the lower class did not coincide with or occur immediately after years with relatively high prices of rye, there was a link between warfare and child mortality.[46] All wars fought between 1726 and

1805 were accompanied by mortality crises among the lower class in Gilze and Rijen.[47] The eight most severe mortality crises among the lower class all occurred during or immediately after wars, with dysentery and typhus being the primary epidemics. Not only were the mortality crises of the upper and middle classes less severe, but they did not coincide with those of the lower class during the eighteenth century.[48]

The rural family reconstitution study carried out for the parish of Penrith in northern England for the years 1600–1800 also reveals social-class distinctions in infant mortality, with the subsistence group (subsistence livestock farmers) having higher infant mortality than the elite class (e.g., gentry, substantial landowners, merchants and clergy) and tradesmen class (e.g., blacksmiths, skinners, butchers, shoemakers, and so on). Scott and Duncan find support for a nutrition-mortality link. The nutrition and diet of the subsistence class of Penrith was suboptimal, particularly during the hungry season and in years of high grain prices.[49]

Other examples from Europe suggest a more complex relationship between social class or occupation and infant and child mortality in particular. In some communities where class-specific mortality differentials have been found, the relationship is not even in the predicted direction. That is, the economically better-off classes do not invariably enjoy lower mortality. Family reconstitution in six early modern, rural German populations indicates that land ownership in premodern Germany did not always translate into survival advantages for children. In Altenesch and in the Krummhörn, survivorship to age fifteen for both sexes was much better for children of workers.[50] A likely explanation for higher male mortality in families with land holdings is that families sought to limit the number of male heirs as well as reduce the rate of inheritance transfers.[51] In terms of female mortality, farmer families were likely responding to socioeconomic circumstances and perhaps trying to limit the number of dowries.[52] In Sweden, Jan Sundin too has found that the relationship between socioeconomic group and mortality contradicts theoretical expectations. During the second half of the eighteenth century, infant mortality was high in most parts of Sweden, but lower on average in the iron foundry industry (among skilled and unskilled workers) than in other more well-to-do socioeconomic groups. Sundin attributes the lower mortality of workers to better child-care practices in the foundry communities. Many foundries employed midwives and sometimes doctors who spread information about the benefits of breastfeeding and hygiene. Sundin suggests that workers were more culturally receptive of child-care advice than other groups, such as farmers, that tended to preserve traditional practices that were often harmful to child survival. Infant-mortality decline, which occurred during the first half of the nineteenth century, was earlier and more rapid in foundry communities than in more prosperous social groups.[53]

Still other studies suggest that the relationship between social class and mortality is uneven in time and place. For example, John Knodel, a member of the European Fertility Project, conducted a detailed analysis of fourteen German village populations in the eighteenth and nineteenth centuries and found little occupational variation in either marital fertility or infant mortality.[54] In terms of infant mortality, Knodel writes: "The fact that all social strata within a village appeared to have shared a more or less common risk of child loss emphasizes the probable role of local or regional infant-feeding customs, common to all classes, as a key determinant of infant mortality."[55] In a similar study of social differences in infant mortality in the Norwegian parish Asker and Baerum in the nineteenth century, Eli Fure finds no evidence of better health care for the foundry workers than for other members of the parish during the mortality transition in nineteenth-century Norway. Fure, following Knodel, suggests that the low overall rate of infant mortality in the parish is best attributed to the existence of cultural breastfeeding practices shared by all inhabitants.[56]

Parish studies by Knodel and Fure illustrate the importance of crosscutting cultural ties (evidenced in shared breastfeeding practices) in leveling out occupational differences in infant mortality at the local level. The studies from Sweden and Altenesch and Krummhörn further demonstrate how infant- and child-mortality experiences are filtered through local conditions and customs. Cultural contingencies of child care and inheritance in Sweden and premodern Germany, respectively, served to reverse the expected health outcomes of social classes. Above all, examples from Germany, Sweden, and Norway illustrate that, in terms of the relationship between class or occupation and demographic outcomes, the European demographic experience is far from being historically or geographically monolithic. While class is clearly an important determinant of a person's life chances in Europe, there is still considerable complexity in the patterning of reproductive behavior in the past.

Local Class Differences in Pretransitional Non-European Countries

While demographic studies on social-class variation in pretransitional populations outside of Europe are few, class distinctions in mortality have been uncovered in pretransitional China.[57] In examining the demographic experiences of lineage groups in the peripheral Tongcheng county of the Lower Yangzi region from 1520–1661, Telford finds that infant-mortality rates in preindustrial Chinese populations varied dramatically by social status.[58] According to Telford, it is the "high-risk" occupations among lower-status families (e.g., peasant farmers, tenants, small traders and craftsmen) that contribute to their higher death rates and lower rates of growth. He cites the long hours of environmental exposure to parasite- and malaria-infested paddy fields among peasant agriculturalists (relative to the educationally qualified elites or gentry class) to account for the higher mortality rates of peasant children. While mortality rates varied by husbands' class standing, the total marital fertility rates of their wives varied little or none at all.[59] Thus, like the situation in historical Europe, there appears to be greater variation in mortality than fertility prior to demographic transition.

Local-level fertility variation prior to transition is not pronounced, but this does not mean that reproductive variation does not exist between regions within countries or across national boundaries. Princeton researchers were well aware of the existence of fertility differentials across such boundaries. Pretransitional studies from countries outside of Europe not only point to fertility variation between regions within countries, but suggest that those differences can be attributed to varying economic circumstances. While information on occupation is not available, there is evidence of a positive relationship between land availability and fertility in pretransitional Thailand[60] and Indonesia.[61] In the case of pretransitional Thailand, the expansion of Thai agriculture is related to political-economic changes in rural areas that opened up new frontiers of cultivation. The beginnings of more extensive frontier settlement in the nineteenth century was linked to a major treaty negotiated between the British and Siamese in 1855, which facilitated the opening up of Thailand's market to British goods and helped make it profitable for investors to ship highly regarded Thai rice abroad.[62] These developments led to a remarkable expansion of the transportation system linking agricultural regions in the surrounding countryside to the core Bangkok area, mostly through canals at the turn of the century. Most of the land in the Thai central plain came under cultivation by 1925. During the 1950s, substantial numbers of young Thai men and women were migrating between rural areas. Most families were leaving the densely settled central region of Thailand in hopes of setting up a new household in sparsely settled frontier areas. Using data from fifty-nine rural provinces in Thailand, Mark Vanlandingham and Charles Hirschman found that couples living at the frontier have higher fertility largely due to the lower costs of family formation at the frontier, the demand for child labor given a shortage of labor in less densely settled areas, and due to the fact that parents will anticipate better prospects for endowing their children with land than will farmers living in more densely settled areas.[63]

The expansion of cultivation in the fertile northern region of Indonesia under Dutch rule also coincided with higher fertility in those areas. David Henley finds that districts in Minhasa, Sulawesi (Indonesia), subject to the greatest degree of compulsory coffee cultivation by the Dutch during the colonial period (1850–1900) also tended to be those in which women had borne the greatest number of children.[64] The primary mechanism appears to be reduced lactational amenorrhea among hard-worked women.[65] While the availability of agricultural land clearly affects fertility levels in preindustrial settings, Vanlandingham and Hirschman observe that, once frontiers have been filled or land prices soar, there is a pattern reversal and fertility begins to decline.[66] This scenario also fits the fertility transition pattern found in Ecuador's Amazonian forest frontier, where a negative relationship between farm size and fertility was reported.[67]

Empirical Revisions and Confirmations

The microdemographic literature confirms that, with few exceptions, reproductive homogeneity characterizes European communities prior to demographic transition, but mortality variation is more pronounced in these same pretransitional populations. Studies from pretransitional Europe and China indicate that class disparities lead to sizable differences in mortality, with poorer classes frequently facing lower survivorship and life expectancy. Microdemographic research on the demographic transition has prompted both revisions and confirmations of some central tenets of demographic transition theory. It is clear that the demographic transition occurred in waves that eventually came to encompass entire populations. However, each wave was induced by political-economic transformations that affected different classes in different ways. The fertility transition may thus be said to be class-specific in terms of its timing and causality. Hence, demographic transition as a local process is better envisioned as a series of transitions rather than a single sweeping event that affected all members of society simultaneously.

Social class or occupation was not an explicit component of most models employed by the European Fertility Project. However, researchers did recognize the role of socially prominent groups as "pioneers" in the fertility transition. Livi-Bacci documents pockets of early fertility decline in the provinces of Europe among a small group of social "forerunners."

These forerunners (e.g., the aristocracies of Milan, Genoa, and Florence; Jewish minorities; and urban populations of Calvinist Geneva and Catholic Rouen) experienced fertility decline earlier—sometimes a century or more before the general population.[68] Microdemographic case studies have similarly confirmed that more privileged classes experience fertility decline earlier than other local class groups. It was the *civil* class in Sicily, the elite groups in Casalecchio, Italy, the landed farmers in England, and the landowning caste/class in India that were the first to curtail their fertility.

The micro-level studies carried out in Sicily, Italy, and India also show that elite classes experienced mortality decline sooner than other local classes, and that mortality decline preceded fertility decline. While it is unclear whether mortality decline occurred prior to fertility decline among social forerunners in European provinces, it does appear that the forerunners had moderate mortality experiences in comparison to other class groups. As Livi-Bacci observes: "Mortality among the forerunners was generally relatively moderate and lower than in the general population."[69] A distinguishing feature of the social groups considered by Livi-Bacci (as opposed to the populations that are the focus of almost all the micro-level studies examined here) is their urban residence. Nevertheless, whatever differences exist in the class structure of urban versus rural societies, the same pattern of moderate mortality is discernable.

It is well known that mortality can influence fertility via both biological and behavioral mechanisms. Infant mortality can reduce the length of the birth interval, either because breastfeeding often ceases with the death of a child or because parents may try to conceive immediately after the loss of a child. As child survivorship improves, a conscious behavioral shift may occur as people come to realize that there is less of a need to replace deceased children. As mentioned previously, improved survivorship has special relevance for landed classes whose status and livelihood are linked to the transmission of undivided patrimony. The Indian case nicely illustrates the precarious balance between family size and land resources in the context of mortality decline. Ultimately, low and stable child mortality means an increase in the number of heirs, which could undermine the class standing of landowning families, unless they adjust their family size accordingly. Das Gupta finds that traditionally landowning families adjusted family size to resources by controlling their sons' marriages (e.g., by postponing their sons' marriages, employing marital celibacy, or through the practice of fraternal polyandry).[70] Hence modern family limitation was entirely compatible with earlier family-limitation strategies, which relied largely on starting behaviors of landowning castes, and often used as security against mortality crises and food shortages.[71]

The preeminence of socioeconomic factors in fertility decline and the fact that mortality decline appears to be an important precursor to falling fertility (among village and town residents studied by microdemographers) lend support to early classic transition theory,[72] which predates the European Fertility Project. Recognition of class and caste-specific differences in fertility and mortality during transition challenges the assumption that women within populations experience homogeneous fertility decline. In short, empirical findings based on microdemographic research seem to contradict the conclusions derived from macrodemographic studies, particularly the European Fertility Project. The class differences uncovered both prior to and at the onset of transition suggest that socioeconomic factors play a pivotal role in shaping human family sizes. This brings us to the fundamental unresolved question as to how to reconcile macrodemographic studies, which emphasize the importance of noneconomic cultural factors in explaining the onset of transition, and microdemographic studies, which reinject economic arguments into explanations of both the onset and pace of transition.

First, it is important to keep in mind that there are ongoing attempts among macrodemographers to determine the precise role of economic factors in fertility decline at the national level. Some analysts of fertility transition have concluded that economic factors may affect the pace of transition, at least in contemporary developing countries, but exert minimal influence otherwise.[73] Secondly, not all demographers concur with the European Fertility Project's emphasis on cultural-ideational factors for explaining fertility transition. For example, Patrick Galloway, Eugene Hammel, and Ronald Lee explain the causes of fertility decline in Prussia (1875–1910) within *Kreise* (an administrative unit similar to a modern census tract, containing some sixty thousand inhabitants) using a very rich and detailed data set and pathbreaking methods (i.e., pooled cross-section and time-series statistical techniques). The authors examine both variation in fertility levels between *Kreise* at particular points in time and change in fertility within *Kreise* over time. Their results show that religion by far accounts for most of the variation in fertility levels between *Kreise*, followed by ethnicity and the proportion of miners. However, their explanation for fertility decline within *Kreise* highlights distinct forces. Their predictive model shows that 80 percent of the decline in marital fertility from 1875 to 1910 is due to structural factors (female labor-force participation, communications and financial services), 15 percent to infant mortality and only 5 percent of the decline is attributable to religious and ethnic variables.[74]

John Brown and Timothy Guinnane come to similar conclusions in their district-level study of rural fertility decline in Bavaria from 1880 to 1910. While the authors do find support for the role of religion in explaining Bavarian fertility decline, with Catholic districts experiencing fertility decline later than non-Catholic districts, their econometric analysis shows that occupation has a striking effect on fertility. Specifically, textile employment (the best proxy for off-farm employment opportunities for women) has a strong negative effect on fertility. The same is true for more direct measures of women's labor opportunities—women's wages. Examination of a third economic variable, farm size, reveals that smaller farms (two to five hectares) that rely on family labor are associated with higher fertility.[75]

In coming to terms with apparent disagreements over the role of economic factors in demographic transition, it is critical to recognize that macro- and microdemographic studies employ distinct methodological approaches. In addition to the quantitative-qualitative divide, there are differences in the conceptual-theoretical and empirical-operational frameworks employed. The economic concepts and measures used by the European Fertility Project are not comparable to those employed in microdemographic studies, and are sometimes not even comparable across macrodemographic studies. Knodel and Van de Walle acknowledge that the socioeconomic indicators used by members of the European Fertility Project to measure the level of socioeconomic development at the onset of fertility decline in Europe and several developing countries (e.g., percentage of the male labor force in agriculture, percent rural, percentage in cities over twenty thousand) were rudimentary: "The measures are crude and suffer from varying degrees of incomparability across countries."[76] However, the authors maintain that because those countries that experienced transition simultaneously displayed such vast differences in their level of social and economic development, the level of socioeconomic development could be ruled out as a necessary precursor for falling fertility.[77]

The most fundamental methodological difference between macro- and microdemographic studies is that they tend to use different units of analysis. Unlike micro-level studies, macro studies focus on broader levels of human social organization. Knodel clearly describes the focus of the European Fertility Project as follows:

The studies sponsored by this project, as well as most studies inspired by it, have been based primarily on macro-level data derived from census and vital statistics reports referring to administrative areas such as nations, provinces, or districts rather than to individuals or individual families per se. Thus, much of the description and analysis of the demographic transition as it took place in the past has been limited to those aspects that can be appropriately addressed by data for such aggregate units.[78]

What applies at the provincial or national level does not necessarily apply to villages, households, or individual women or men. It is imperative to distinguish units of analysis and observation when constructing explanations of demographic diversity and change. If researchers are investigating demographic behavior at different spatial or temporal scales, then they are in effect explicating different features of reproductive behavior, which means that concurrence of observation is not to be expected. Social forces that take precedence at the regional or national level and over broad stretches of time might be different than those operating within local communities at shorter time scales.

For example, imagine a hypothetical village located in a Flemish area of Belgium, where all of the local residents speak Flemish, understand French, and are Catholic. Suppose that in spite of the fact that village residents are homogeneous with respect to language and religion, women still show tremendous diversity in their completed family sizes. Now, it is highly unlikely that researchers would attribute those local fertility differentials to the constant variables of language or religion. This may seem so obvious that it need not be mentioned—it is part of the logic of experimental control. However, it leads us to appreciate that, in order to determine whether or not research findings are truly contradictory or incompatible, we must pay closer attention to the scale of investigation in time and space. At different scales, different social facts may be relevant to the explanation of demographic behavior. Attention to scale is implicit in demographic studies, as researchers routinely distinguish between the causes/consequences of inter- and intrapopulation/intrasocietal/intracultural variation in human fertility. However, greater conceptual and empirical rigor is needed in specifying the spatiotemporal units of analysis and observation in demographic research.

The demographic studies undertaken in Prussia and Bavaria do not directly challenge the findings of the European Fertility Project, particularly those of Knodel. Both studies in the German Kingdom were undertaken at levels of analysis finer than provincial units. The Prussian *Kreise* is "one-fifteenth the size of the typical unit of analysis used in the European Fertility Project."[79] Similarly, the analysis of Bavaria by Brown and Guinnane relies on a set of rural and urban districts with more detail (finer grain and extent) than the units used by the European Fertility Project.[80] However, other important questions have been raised about the findings of the European Fertility Project, particularly the need for more varied and less simplified measures of economic influences, and for recognition that findings from Western Europe may not coincide with macro studies from other geographic regions and continents.[81]

Demographers are increasingly acknowledging the importance of spatial and temporal scale in interpreting fertility variation and change. Karen Mason was one of the first demographers to suggest that our understanding of fertility transitions needs to be guided by an awareness of temporal scale. On a millennial time scale, theoretical explanations for global fertility decline focus on why the transition occurred during the last two hundred years. Yet, such theories may not necessarily answer questions about why fertility transition began in a particular locale in one decade versus another.[82] Similarly, Potter, Schmertmann and Cavenaghi observe that cross-sectional studies of fertility and mortality highlight different patterns and processes than longitudinal studies: "incorporating temporal and spatial information can lead to different inferences about fertility's relationship to covariates."[83] However, distinctions of temporal scale are more readily acknowledged than those of spatial scale. That is, there is no clear recognition among researchers that conceptual-empirical conclusions derived from their finer-scale studies may not be strictly comparable to those obtained from more macro studies that rely on broader geographic units (such as those considered by the European Fertility Project). Instead, researchers frequently suggest that their finer-scale studies are superior to and contradict findings based on larger geographic units. There is considerable discomfort and mistrust of studies involving larger-level units (countries and provinces).

For example, Potter, Schmertmann, and Cavenaghi write: "The difficulty with the former is that they are plagued by vast amounts of unmeasured heterogeneity—countries clearly vary one from another in myriad aspects that are not captured by the available indicators."[84] Brown and Guinnane make a similar point: "the Princeton Project's large units masked considerable internal heterogeneity."[85] Galloway, Hammel, and Lee also invoke scale only to insist on the primacy of finer units of analysis:

Nearly all the conclusions from the Princeton European Fertility Project are based on studies in which larger units of analysis were used. These were often called provinces, which in Prussia correspond to *Regierungsbezirke*, the next higher administrative level above the *Kreise*. These units may, in fact, be too large, and in the case of Germany, and of Prussian data in particular, analysis of such highly aggregated units can lead to unwarranted conclusions. Knodel, Richards, Lesthaeghe and Wilson, and Coale and Watkins used 30 *Regierungsbezirke* as units of analysis when working with Prussia, while we shall use 407 *Kreise*.[86]

The unease with which social scientists approach highly aggregated analyses parallels concerns over reductionism, except here the concern lies not in reducing the whole to its parts, but in subsuming parts to the whole, or wholism. It seems to me that sociodemographic phenomena can be studied at a variety of scales without resorting to reductionism or wholism. A scalar approach recognizes nested realities. (For example, global life expectancy at birth may be 64.5 years; but, at a finer regional level, in sub-Saharan Africa, where the HIV epidemic is most prevalent, life expectancy at birth is less than thirty-five years.) The important point is to note that pattern and process, as well as their relationship, may change with temporal *and* spatial scale. When examining broader levels of human social organization or looking from the top down, broader levels act as "wholes," but when looking from the bottom up, finer levels in the hierarchy act as "parts." This is what hierarchy theorists refer to as the "Janus-faced" nature of subsystems at each level within a hierarchy.[87]

It is clear from microdemographic case studies that the argument for reproductive homogeneity at the local level in state-level societies (i.e., several European countries, Nepal, and India) is untenable. Behavioral variation within local communities, according to class/caste or occupation, is evident, which seriously challenges the notion of homogenous fertility decline at the local community level. However, this does not mean that regional and cultural-linguistic factors are not important at broader scales of investigation. Microdemographic studies are bound by their own limitations. Such studies do not generally examine multiple spatial scales simultaneously or seek to determine whether demographic variation within communities exceeds variation between communities or larger aggregates such as provinces and nations. Researchers must be careful not to overstate the findings of either macro- or micro-level research. The principal error in reasoning that lies at the base of homogenous fertility-decline arguments is the ecological fallacy, or assuming that when relationships are found among aggregate data, these relationships will also be found among individuals, households, and localities. Macrodemographic researchers are more vulnerable to the ecological fallacy, whereas microdemographers are more prone to the individualistic fallacy—the practice of generalizing from individual behavior to aggregate relationships. Hence, it would be equally erroneous for microdemographers to "scale up" by generalizing from village and town studies to provinces and nations (in effect heralding class or a similar factor as "the master key" that explains demographic variation at both finer *and* broader scales).

Conclusion

The role of socioeconomic factors, particularly class inequality, in understanding social variation in human family sizes, and infant and child mortality is a central focus of contemporary microdemographic inquiry in the social sciences. A growing body of research over the last few decades has found that social stratification, related to both class and caste, is crucial to understanding variation in microdemographic behavior during the demographic transition in parts of Europe and Asia. Evidence of local heterogeneity in the transitional experiences of European and non-European societies seriously challenges notions of local reproductive homogeneity often inferred from macrodemographic studies. It is problematic to infer homogeneous fertility decline at the local level in studies largely conducted at higher levels of aggregation and longer time frames (such as those initiated or inspired by the Princeton European Fertility Project).

Studies that do not overlap in terms of units of analysis or geographical-historical context should not necessarily be expected to coincide in their conclusions about demographic behavior. In this light, it is more appropriate to view such studies as distinct, and perhaps even complementary, as opposed to competing or incompatible. Shifting scales may require a shift in our conceptual model, which, in turn, implies recognition of multiple levels of causality in the explanation of demographic phenomena. Social class or occupation is a critical part of a general explanation for both the timing and pace of fertility decline at the local level. However, class-specific microfertility differentials in pretransitional (as opposed to transitional) societies are minimal—the overall pattern is one of reproductive uniformity. While class differences in mortality prior to transition are apparent, the patterning of mortality at the local level is still complex. The absence of class-specific infant-mortality differentials in several European communities points to the influence of local sociocultural institutions and practices that transcend class boundaries. Under unique cultural-historical circumstances, class advantage can even confer survival disadvantages. Such exceptions prompt us to more carefully investigate the contexts and mechanisms underlying class differences in demographic behavior at different stages of transition.

Historical exceptions from Europe lend support to Joachim Vogel and Töres Theorell's observation that different institutions and practices can be used to address inequalities in health. In the contemporary context, some countries (modern Sweden and Finland) rely predominantly on the welfare state, with its taxation and borrowing powers, to monitor the transfer and distribution of income. Others (e.g., the modern United States and United Kingdom) rely mostly on the labor market (employers) for welfare distribution.[88] Although the authors downplay the effectiveness of the family in reducing the level of inequality in contemporary European nations, the studies reviewed here (historical Sweden, Germany, and Norway) as well as those in the next chapter demonstrate that family ties, community norms, and cultural practices can modify or overstep the initial wealth distribution to produce health equalities. Continuing to specify the conditions under which class differences do not translate into differences in reproduction and survivorship is critical to identifying alternative health systems. The microdemographic studies reviewed here also reinforce the need for a broader political-economic analysis in order to understand microreproductive behavior. While demographers are likely to continue to debate the relative importance of socioeconomic versus cultural factors in explaining demographic differentials in time and space, there is more than a little irony in the fact that macrodemographers, many of whom are economic demographers, have come to champion the role of culture in demographic explanation, whereas microdemographers, many of whom are cultural anthropologists, have reinstated an economic calculus in the explanation of demographic transitions.

8

Demography on the Nomadic Periphery

Chapter 7 documents the presence of social-class, caste, and occupational variation in demographic behavior in different parts of Europe, Asia, and Latin America during transition. The question that remains unclear is whether or not similar forms of local socioeconomic differentiation shape the demographic experiences of less stratified peoples peripheral to state control, particularly nomadic groups. It is well known that humankind has lived out most of its history in nomadic bands or tribes whose very existence is threatened by the ascendancy of Western capitalist society. The few tribal societies that remain today occupy peripheral spaces within and between nation-state boundaries, although it must be borne in mind that there is considerable diversity in the type and character of social interactions between these communities and broader rural and urban industrial systems. In this chapter, I review empirical-interpretive accounts of sociodemographic inequality in tribal pastoralist and hunting-gathering economies. Even though we have little information on the histories of many small-scale nomadic societies—most of the demographic studies examined here are twentieth-century accounts—all patterns of social interaction are located in time and space. Hence, my emphasis is on a time-geography of interaction that attempts to move away from reified accounts of "primitive" peoples as "static," "unchanging," and "isolated."

Sociality, Mortality, and Health in Nomadic Societies

Daniel Bradburd has argued that because today's nomadic populations are integrated into regional, national, and global systems, "we should therefore expect nomadic societies to show many of the same features of the transition to capitalism as other agrarian (previously) precapitalist systems."[1] Indeed, in his research among Komachi pastoralists of Iran, Bradburd found emergent class distinctions between elite employer-shepherds, who rely on hired labor for herding, and their hired shepherd employees.[2] In terms of

class differentials in demographic behavior, census data on Komachi pastoralists from Iran reveals that, on average, 22.3 percent of the children born
to hired shepherd families died in childhood, compared to only 15.6 percent
in employer-shepherd families.[3]

Philip Salzman, however, cautions that classes in pastoral societies are
largely found among peasant pastoralists, who through peasantization processes have experienced reduced political autonomy or increased state encapsulation, as well as greater involvement in national and international
exchange markets.[4] Pastoralists like the Baluch,[5] Yomut Turkmen,[6] and
Bedouin Arabs[7] are largely egalitarian, Salzman argues, because they are
located in peripheral geographic areas far removed from effective state control (that is until recently). Hence, such pastoralists continue to invoke their
segmentary organization for defense and protection.[8] The documentation
of mortality differentials is essential to evaluating theoretical arguments of
nonegalitarianism. It would be difficult to defend arguments of sociopolitical egalitarianism if vast differences in mortality between social groups were
uncovered.[9] Class, racial, and other social disparities in morbidity and mortality help us identify structural violence and inequalities. Disease, illness
and injury, which often lead to premature death and short life expectancy,
are among the most important indicators of social suffering. While death
statistics based on numbers cannot reveal the agony of human suffering,
particularly in extreme situations like the Native American holocaust,[10] nu-
merical figures can put such suffering into sharp focus. If differential morbidity and mortality were not consequences of social inequalities of class,
race/ethnicity, gender, and nationality, then these social facts would lose
much of their relevance, save for identity politics.

Bedouin agropastoralists in the Bekaa Valley have clearly been implicated
in peasantization processes over the last half century. Most notably, since
the beginning of agricultural and infrastructural development under the
French Mandate, the nomadic movements of tribes have been increasingly
circumscribed and controlled by the state. The mechanization of transport
in the mid-1960s accelerated sedentarization and villagization processes in
Bedouin society. Such peasantization processes have been accompanied in
many parts of the world by class stratification.[11] My research among Bedouins shows that distinct economic groups (pastoralists, sharecroppers, and
wage laborers) do not have their own demographic regimes. Even as Bedouin nomadic movements were increasingly confined by the demarcation
of state boundaries and their grazing lands were encroached upon by land
privatization and agricultural expansion, Bedouins continue to engage in
social practices within their own communities that undercut class stratifi-

cation. Coercive state power is rarely absolute. Power, like other structural features of social life, must be analyzed as involving "reproduced relations of autonomy and dependence."[12] Aside from differentials of power and their contestation, it is also important to recognize that actors' knowledgeability about the conditions or outcomes of social episodes is always bounded. One of the implications of this is that actions often have unintended consequences. For example, as Bedouins sold their livestock to purchase land for residence, many did not anticipate that economic subordination would be one of the long-term implications of their actions.

While some anthropologists have suggested that egalitarianism in pastoral societies is a myth,[13] recent discussions have clarified that these disagreements stem, in part, from different definitions of egalitarianism. If social theorists define egalitarianism on the basis of economic inequality, then most pastoral societies are inegalitarian. However, Salzman[14] and Irons[15] have pointed out that economic inequality oscillates considerably in pastoral societies. Salzman defines egalitarianism on the basis of sociopolitical organization, not economic inequality. Egalitarian societies can be defined as societies characterized by decentralization, generalized participation in violence and the enforcement of social order, the absence of specialized institutions or a permanent class of rulers or warriors, and individual and democratic decision-making. Bedouin tribes in the Middle East and North Africa are considered among the more egalitarian, decentralized of segmentary tribes known to humanity. In addition to the Bekaa Bedouin, the Rwala Bedouin of Arabia,[16] the Al Murrah Bedouin of the Empty Quarter (Saudi Arabia),[17] the Sanusi Bedouin of Cyrenaica (Libya),[18] the Hadramaut Bedouin of Yemen,[19] and even the Awlad 'Ali Bedouin of Egypt[20] have been described as politically egalitarian.

The more pressing question is: under what cultural-historical and ecological conditions are egalitarian societies found? Irons proposes that egalitarianism is not due to the absence of economic inequality per se, but the absence of economic inequality over the long term. Irons explains how in Yomut society, economic inequality in the form of patrimony does not predict wealth at the time of his survey. Rather, livestock wealth fluctuates enormously, and wealth differences largely even out through time—a situation that helps explain Yomut society's egalitarianism. This leads Irons to suggest that social stratification may be more likely in contexts where economic inequality shows long-term structural effects.[21] Following Irons, I chose to examine the effects of inheritance at marriage (i.e., indirect and direct dowries combined) on wealth in the means of production at the time of the survey (controlling for marriage duration). Because my findings suggest that inheritance positively correlates with wealth ownership at the time of the survey, I was unable to account for egalitarianism using Irons's hypothesis.

Thomas Barfield provides an alternative geographical-historical explanation for egalitarianism/hierarchy among Middle Eastern tribes. Barfield explains how egalitarian lineage structures have long been indigenous to the region and are related to historical-political geography and cultural ecology. Arabian tribes inhabit a region with a more limited set of resources that could support only relatively weak military forces. Their state political structures were more unstable and subject to regular collapse. Tribes in the Middle East were on more even terms when dealing with states, enjoyed greater autonomy, and were egalitarian in terms of both their kinship structure and cultural ideology. While states in the Middle East have traditionally been divided into small regional states, Turco-Mongolian tribes lived in a region that was under the control of great empires. As a result, Turco-Mongolian tribal systems are more hierarchical in their kinship and political organization, with hundreds of thousands of people under the authority of powerful khans.[22] Egalitarian tribes and small regional states appear to co-occur in the Middle East. Classlike distinctions and class-specific demographic differentials may depend more on political geography than strictly economic forces. Social-class hierarchies are a question of scale. In the Bekaa Valley, Lebanon, the markers of class are not visible within Bedouin communities, but distinguish Bedouin, peasant, and city dweller from one another.

Class or classlike divisions in the Middle East have been uncovered among several pastoral groups, including the Komachi in south-central Iran,[23] the Qashqa'i in southwest Iran,[24] and the Lurs of Pish-e Kuh Luristan in west Iran.[25] With the exception of Komachi pastoralists in Iran, there is a lack of demographic evidence to assess whether or not reported classlike distinctions have given rise to demographic differentials. Salzman has argued, in a manner similar to Barfield, that tribes fully integrated into the lowest levels of state systems and that have no access to coercive resources with which to defend their interests are more centralized and less segmentary in their organization.[26] Such pastoralists are referred to as "peasant pastoralists"—pastoralists who lack an internal political structure, political leaders, or a sense of tribal unity.[27] Are the Bekaa Bedouin best seen as peasant pastoralists?[28] I believe that the answer is no. Peasantization of the Bedouin is not complete. The Bedouin of the Bekaa are in a transitional phase in their history. Their agropastoral economy is highly peasantized. Pastoralism in particular has undergone fundamental transformations, with its modern reliance on trucks, purchased feed, and overall sedentary pattern. Nevertheless, internally, there is neither recognized ranking among tribes nor cultural devaluation of different tribes. In spite of their experiences with dispossession under peasantization (loss of traditional land base and water for grazing), Bekaa Bedouins have maintained a degree of political autonomy, communal solidarity, and health equity.[29] Perhaps most importantly, unlike the situation among Komachi pastoralists of Iran, where class conflict stems from the exploitative economic relationship between employer-shepherds and their hired shepherd employees,[30] Lebanese Bedouin rely on family labor for herding. Following Bradburd's reasoning, the socioeconomic conditions necessary for class exploitation are absent and better sought elsewhere, namely in the relationship between Lebanese Bedouin pastoralists and hired Syrian Bedouin shepherds—an economic arrangement more common in the past.

Anthropological studies on nomadic pastoral communities outside the Middle East can also be used to address questions about social-class disparities in health in time and space. Numerous studies point to the detrimental social and economic impacts of pastoral sedentarization and commoditization processes, including poorer nutrition and a lack of adequate housing and drinking water; however, sedentary groups seem to have access to better health care.[31] In terms of socioeconomic differentiation at the local level, Elliot Fratkin, Eric Roth, and Martha Nathan found no evidence of inequalities in child health and nutritional status among Rendille pastoralists of northern Kenya. The authors attribute this to the fact that children from livestock-poor families receive approximately the same amount of milk as children from livestock-rich families.[32] Hence sharing of milk animals and milk itself helps negate livestock-ownership differences.

Similarly, in his evaluation of the nutritional consequences of wealth differentials among the Datoga pastoralists of northern Tanzania, Dan Sellen found little evidence of social inequality in child health. Although considerable variation in household wealth was apparent, no health benefits (in terms of average growth performance) were found among young children in relatively wealthy households.[33] In contrast, Kel Tamasheq (Tuareg) nomadic herders from the West African Sahel show pronounced health inequities. Tuareg society is very hierarchical, with an intricate class system that includes *iklan* (slaves) and richer high-status *illelan* (free people) for whom many of the former group work. Analyses reveal substantial mortality differences by social class for both children and adults. Although increasing numbers of *iklan* (slaves) were freed in the 1950s, Sara Randall reports that at the time of the surveys in the early 1980s, social class was still a good indicator of household wealth, with some *iklan* continuing to live in virtual slavery.[34]

While it is clear that pastoral societies are diverse, claims that egalitarianism within those societies is a myth are not substantiated. Future demographic research is needed to understand the patterning of social inequalities within and between pastoral communities, but the Bekaa Bedouin, Rendille, and Datoga cases point to a high degree of health parity at the local level. The same appears to be true for nomadic foraging groups, but, unfortunately, studies on social inequality in health within foraging communities are infrequently related to analytical interpretations of pastoralist, agrarian, and urban ethnic communities. Most of the demographic studies on foragers have been conducted by biodemographers with distinct theoretical orientations and methodologies. Biodemographic research on nomadic peoples, particularly foragers, has focused less on micro-level class or economic distinctions and more on the impact of broader economic modes of subsistence on infant and child mortality. Aggregated analyses performed by Dan Sellen and Ruth Mace—using the Human Relations Area Files (HRAF) and other anthropological sources—indicate a positive association between dependence on extractive modes of subsistence (hunting, gathering, and fishing) and total child mortality.[35] However, the same cross-cultural analyses indicate that infant-mortality rates do not vary with subsistence activity. Thus, the authors conclude that it is problematic to argue that the availability of easily digestible, nutrient-rich weaning foods (i.e., dairy or cereal products) in pastoral and agricultural economies substantially reduces infant mortality. Instead, it is more likely that the protective effects of continued breastfeeding throughout the first year of life—believed to be omnipresent in traditional societies—served to reduce the variance in infant mortality across subsistence economies.[36]

Renee Pennington has also looked at how heightened involvement in agriculture among foraging groups impacts infant and child mortality. Pennington argues that the decline in early mortality among Ju/'hoansi children is due to changes that accompanied sedentism, namely increased caloric intakes as a result of greater access to domesticated-animal milk from Herero cattle posts.[37] Pennington goes beyond this to propose that access to cow's or other milk as well as other high-protein weaning foods helps to explain much of the variation in child-mortality rates across world regions. If we include life-table estimates of Bedouin mortality alongside infant- and child-mortality rates compiled by Pennington for seven peripheral societies,[38] the data shows that infant mortality ranges from a low of .05 among the Bedouin and .06 among recently born Herero of Botswana to a high of .24 among an ethnically mixed population of Mandinka and Jola in the Gambia. The lowest early-childhood-mortality rates, .02, are found among the Bedouin and among the most recently born cohort of Herero children (.03). The highest childhood-mortality rates are found among Delta Fulani in Mali, where .36 of children reaching the age of one die before they turn five. It does appear that the two groups (Herero and Bedouin) with the lowest infant- and child-mortality rates are also those that have access to milk and milk products as well as protein-rich weaning foods. Also important in understanding lower mortality among Bedouin is the presence of clinics and hospitals in the Bekaa that provide safe birthing practices and maternal health services. Younger Bedouin women are increasingly having their children in a hospital. Even older women, who mostly reported giving birth at home, did so with the assistance of a peasant midwife or an older Bedouin woman with previous childbirth delivery experience.

Biodemographic studies that compare mortality profiles across economic modes of subsistence do little to address questions about inequality between individuals and groups within hunting-gathering economies. With that said, questions about social inequality have been central to the Great Kalahari debate on foragers, which is half a century old. On one side of the debate are the "traditionalists," led by Richard Lee and the Harvard Kalahari Group, who regard the Ju/'hoansi studied between 1950 and 1965 as relatively autonomous and affluent hunter-gatherers. On the other side are the "revisionists," led by Edwin Wilmsen (author of *Land Filled with Flies: A Political Economy of the Kalahari*), who see the Ju/'hoansi and other hunter-gatherers like them as victims of a capitalist world economy—a marginalized and dispossessed rural proletariat.[39] One of the underlying assumptions questioned by the revisionists is the idea of modern-day foragers as "living fossils" whose lifeways can provide insights into prehistoric Paleolithic hunting-gathering peoples. Instead, hunter-gatherer revisionists argued that Holocene hunter-gatherer societies did not live in isolation from surrounding state societies, but had long histories of trade and interaction with farming and herding peoples (often engaging in part-time cultivation themselves) and thus depended on the outside world for survival.[40] It is clear that hunter-gatherers today rarely if ever obtain all of their food from hunting and gathering, but rely on agriculture and agropastoralism, government welfare, and wage labor.[41] There is increasing archaeological evidence suggestive of nonegalitarian relations (beyond those of age and gender) among prehistoric hunter-gatherers who were more sedentary, lived in densely populated communities, and engaged in large-scale food storage.[42] However, only a few ethnographic examples of nonegalitarian foragers have been identified, including Indians of North America's Northwest Coast, the Ainu of Japan, and the Calusa of Florida.[43]

One of the dangers with the foraging debate (and other debates, for that matter) is that as the lines get more firmly drawn and polarization sets in, one or both sides can slip into universalizing and essentializing arguments. Revisionists are more prone to see structures of domination as one-way and absolute. The agency of foraging peoples is almost completely erased. From this perspective, foragers are regarded as perfect victims, making it imperative to dismiss accounts of hunter-gatherers as "fiercely egalitarian."[44] Traditionalists, on the other hand, can come across as wide-eyed romantics who see foragers as timeless "relics"—static and unchanging in their primitive majesty. With such polarized positions, one is hard-pressed to find either viewpoint appealing. The foraging debate also reflects the need to look more closely at how social relations of domination are geographically and historically patterned. Social divisions of class, ethnicity, and gender need to be situated in their time-space contexts. The convergence of geographic divisions and social inequalities is one of the contextual features of social life. Asymmetries of power are often spatially marked. You change the geographic/historic scale and you change the context of social interactions and hierarchical organization. This is nicely illustrated using Wilmsen's political-economic study of the Kalahari.

Wilmsen shows how groups like the Tswana on the southern and eastern fringes of the Kalahari, who had established agropastoral incipient states, or chiefdoms, by the mid-eighteenth century, were able to consolidate their wealth and expand their power over other Kalahari peoples during the course of the nineteenth century. It was the colonial trader boom that instigated a new level of competition between different Tswana groups. Tswana were successful in recruiting different peoples into their polities, and those groups whose land sat astride the most profitable European trade routes benefited most. An interesting insight to emerge from Wilmsen's study is the explication of isolation as less a matter of ecology than of political geography and political economy/political ecology.[45]

When ethnographers first encountered Kalahari foragers, they did so in the aftermath of a colonial bust phase that was preceded by an economic boom phase in the 1890s. The colonial downturn coincided with the collapse of the ivory/feather trade and the onset of rinderpest, which resulted in the disappearance of most cattle and wild ungulates of southern Africa. Many European settler-traders and hunters returned home, some with sizable fortunes, leaving the San inhabitants to etch out a living on nuts and berries and wild herds that had not been exterminated by white colonists. In brief, isolation and remoteness in the region were generated by the collapse of merchant capital. With the collapse of hunting, ivory subsided and cattle emerged as the main source of wealth in the Kalahari.[46] In an expanding cattle economy, which was marked by the capitalization of land and labor, displaced and dispossessed San became a surplus labor pool. Some were able to achieve a measure of security by finding a cattle-post position, a few San families managed to accumulate small herds of their own, and others turned to the diamond mines for work. However, most San who were either unable or unwilling to participate in the exploitative regional economies retreated to marginal ecological zones of the Kalahari to engage in foraging.[47] Prior to European incursions, social relations were marked more by reciprocity and less by exploitation. During the first half of the nineteenth century, San-speaking peoples maintained a high degree of autonomy and were far removed from European trade routes in southern Africa. Social relations between San and Herero were both fluid and diverse at this time.[48] Similarly, San and Tswana social formations showed little economic or status differentiation in the early eighteenth century.[49]

Wilmsen is able to make sense of the contemporary social positioning of San-speaking peoples by tracing their consolidation into an underclass within colonial economies of the nineteenth and twentieth centuries. Wilmsen also documents inequities in livestock ownership among twentieth-century San speakers. Less than one-third of households in a language group own cattle and less than 10 percent of households own more than half of all animals contained within their group—a pattern similar to that of rural households in Botswana.[50] Yet, there is little information on whether these internal wealth differences translate into health differentials. As we have seen from ethnographic examples in foraging and pastoral societies, practices of food sharing, reciprocity, and redistribution can even out wealth differences. San-speaking Zhu, classified as pastoralists and independent, are 10 percent heavier than foragers, and their weight tends to fluctuate less seasonally.[51] It thus appears that there are minor health advantages for Zhu and other San-speaking peoples with access to cattle in rural Botswana. Given the absence of more detailed information on internal health disparities among Zhu and other San-speaking communities and given historical and contemporary ethnographic accounts of reciprocal social relations in various communities, no firm conclusions can be drawn with respect to internal stratification or internal social disparities in health. The regional patterning and character of social divisions needs to be further investigated.

Some interpret arguments of egalitarianism as evidence of romanticization of "primitive" peoples prompted by the colonial encounter. Anthropologists are suspicious of arguments in support of egalitarianism because they are seen as bordering on naïve romanticism. Careful not to take a position that may be construed as "biased" or too "soft" on natives, anthropologists of various theoretical persuasions are quick to produce evidence of inequality (no matter how puny) to demonstrate that egalitarianism is a myth and inequality universal. To paraphrase the comments of one cultural anthropologist: "The natives are just as shitty [i.e., classist, racist, and sexist] as we are!" We should be wary of cultural projections (especially when they emanate from anthropologists). Extreme postmodern cynicism is not corrective of romanticism. Besides, if inequality is universal, then why bother with sociohistorical analysis at all? Other anthropologists I have spoken to on the matter do not want to be perceived as either native-enthusiasts or native-detractors, so they opt for the safe middle ground. Their position is that there are equalities and inequalities—a little of this and a little of that. This muddled middle position is not much of an improvement. In fact, it appears to fit the definition of the logical fallacy known as *argumentum ad temperantiam*, or "argument to moderation." An appeal to moderation is based on the false assumption that a middle-ground position always provides the "truth" about ourselves and our social worlds.[52]

We must acknowledge the romanticized Western conception of the "noble savage" uncorrupted by the temptations of civilization. Careful examination of Euramerican fascination with the "primitive" reveals asymmetrical and conflicting interests of power. Native cultures and identities have emerged as new sites of appropriation that recollect white colonization of Indian lands and wealth.[53] The practice of "going native" embraced by Euramericans is more concerned with preserving *what is believed to be* Indian culture rather than any concern for Indians themselves. Native knowledge is largely valued for the spiritual and economic benefits it provides to white society.[54] Contact with the "primitive" gives Westerners a temporary release from restrictive social norms; it "can trigger self-transformation and the experience of dissolved hierarchies and boundaries."[55] As anthropologists working in tribal communities, we must be conscious of the relationship between power and representation, particularly when evaluating evidence of egalitarianism. Through our studies on pastoral, foraging, and peasant communities, we must continue to clarify and refine not only what egalitarianism means, but what it does not mean. Egalitarianism is not a euphemism for meekness, passivity, or childish innocence. Egalitarian does not imply unvarying. And it certainly does not denote "inferior" or "less evolved."

Neither egalitarianism nor class stratification can be taken as givens. Embracing a monolithic and transhistorical concept of "class" is not an antidote to homogenous and derogatory classifications of southern African and other colonized peoples invented by the powerful. Colonial violence and subjugation at one level does not necessarily imply asymmetrical relations of power at all levels of human social organization in time and space. To suggest that egalitarianism among hunter-gatherers is simply a byproduct of colonial subjugation—the condition and consolation of the loser—is not only demeaning of foraging peoples, but is conceptually flawed. Archaeologist Robert Kelly describes how the maintenance of an egalitarian social order requires an ongoing commitment on the part of individual members:

> In fact, there is always a tendency for some individuals to attempt to lord it over others. In response, egalitarian hunter-gatherers have developed a variety of ways to level individuals—to "cool their hearts" as the Ju/'hoansi say. Humor is used to belittle the successful hunter; wives use sexual humor to keep a husband in line; and gambling, accusations of stinginess, or demand sharing maintain a constant circulation of goods and prevent hoarding . . . Sharing insures future reciprocity. But in so doing, sharing creates tension as it establishes debts and proclaims differences in ability. The self-effacing behavior of foragers such as the Ju/'hoansi makes sharing easier. A hunter who acknowledges his worthlessness while dropping a fat antelope by the hearth relieves tension created by sharing. The result is not a group of disgruntled would-be misers and dictators, but individuals who are assertively egalitarian, who live a life in which the open hoarding of goods or the imposition of one's will upon another is at odds with cultural norms.[56]

An egalitarian social order is constituted in and through the practices of individuals. Individuals are actively involved in reproducing social life by interpreting and acting upon social norms. Sharing is not automatic or tension-free. Rather, sharing requires social effort and must continuously be renegotiated and put into practice.

Sometimes researchers who posit enduring forms of social inequality (reproduced relations of rank or stratification) among hunter-gatherers are specifically referring to gender inequality, in which case it is necessary to make explicit whether those gender hierarchies refer to inter- or intragender encounters. While some anthropologists have argued that male-on-female dominance is universal, ethnographic studies have described gender relations among hunter-gatherers, such as the Ju/'hoansi, Mbuti, Agta, Batak, Paliyans, and Chipewyans, as nonhierarchical.[57] Demographic evidence on gender disparities in health would help clarify some of the different challenges men and women face in foraging societies. Some gender differences in mortality have been identified among Ju/'hoansi men and women between 1963 and 1973. During this period, women had a higher probability of death in the fifteen to fifty-nine and sixty-plus age groups, whereas men experienced more deaths in the zero to fourteen age group.[58] Gender differences in health have also been found among Ache foragers living south of the Amazon tropical forest in the Alto Parana area of eastern Paraguay. Infant survival was higher for Ache men in the forest period, whereas infant survival was higher for Ache women during the reservation period (1978–1993). In both the forest and reservation periods, boys show slightly higher survivorship in childhood, but women have higher survivorship later in life.[59]

The health gap between contemporary foragers and neighboring pastoral and agrarian communities in southern African is not widely disputed. The average life expectancy of Ju/'hoansi living in the Dobe area (on the border between Botswana and Namibia) in the 1960s and 1970s was 34.57 years.[60] Many contemporary hunter-gatherers are chronically undernourished and vulnerable to periodic and seasonal famines.[61] Thus, it would be irresponsible not to acknowledge demographic differentiation between modern foraging peoples and urban as well as rural folks in rich countries. Explicating how class and other relations of power implicated in health inequities are constituted across time-space can help clarify the structural contours of class in global North and South countries.

Fertility in Nomadic Societies

The abundance of demographic evidence documenting class differences in the onset and pace of fertility transition (particularly in Europe) leads us to ask whether class plays a similar role in explaining fertility variation and change in nomadic societies. While anthropological demographic studies of nomadic groups undergoing fertility transition are lacking, it is possible to examine the reproductive experiences of pretransition nomadic groups to determine whether or not they tell a familiar story of socioeconomic differentiation in microfertility behavior. To determine the extent of local variation in fertility, I decided to examine the fertility distributions of less stratified, nomadic/seminomadic societies, including the Bekaa Bedouin. Table 8.1 shows the distribution of age-specific cumulative fertility (the number of live births ever produced by an individual of any specified age) among women in seven nomadic communities. These communities were not randomly selected but were chosen because they represent nomadic

Table 8.1. The distribution of fertility among seven nomadic societies (classified by five-year age groups)

Age	Bekaa Bedouin			Ganj		
	No.	Mean	VAR	No.	Mean	VAR
15–19	13	1.46	1.94			
20–24	29	2.97	3.82			
25–29	43	3.60	3.25			
30–34	55	5.71	7.14			
35–39	39	7.18	5.41			
40–44	32	8.66	7.52			
45–49	39	8.51	11.05	15	4.1	6.64
50–54	26	9.96	3.48	12	4.2	4.15
55–59	5	11.6	4.30	9	5.0	4.00
60+				26	5.15	5.66

Age	Turkana Northwest Kenya			Ache			Aka Pygmies		
	No.	Mean	VAR	No.	Mean	VAR	No.	Mean	VAR
15–19									
20–24									
25–29									
30–34									
35–39									
40–44	165	6.1	5.29				34	6.23	5.20
45–49									
50–54				42	7.67	5.50			
55–59									
60+									

Sources for non-Bedouin groups: Ganj: Wood, Johnson and Campbell 1985; !Kung: Howell 2000; Fulbe: Marriott 1993; Turkana: Little and Leslie 1999; Ache: Hill and Hurtado 1996; and Aka Pygmies: Hewlett 1988.

societies for whom high-quality demographic data are available. Because evidence of recent fertility decline is only found among the Bedouin, such data can only be used to address questions of within-population variation prior to fertility transition.

The distributions of women's fertility show a high degree of uniformity in the reproductive experiences of women. Although the groups shown in table 8.1 have different levels of fertility, with the Bedouin having the highest and the Ganj the lowest weighted mean cumulative fertility of women

!Kung (Ju/'Hoansi)			Delta Fulbe		
No.	Mean	VAR	No.	Mean	VAR
29	0				
50	.26	.28	42	2.0	1.44
31	1.13	1.18	37	3.8	3.24
58	3.07	2.70	25	6.0	4.84
23	4.22	4.72	12	6.5	6.76
29	4.66	5.82	6	5.5	7.84
14	4.71	2.53			
8	3.87	2.70			
17	4.00	2.75			
23	3.57	2.98			

over forty, they are similar in that the variance in female cumulative fertility is roughly equal to the mean for each age. This means that women within each society are surprisingly uniform in their reproductive experiences, both among themselves (as shown by their low variances) and with respect to age (as shown by the linear increase in their cumulative fertility).[62] The fact that the sample distributions in table 8.1 are best described by a Poisson distribution (which have a variance equal to or slightly less than the mean)[63] indicates that there is similarity with respect to age in these samples, and that there are minimal systematic differences among women in their total fertility.[64] In other words, women who survive to the end of the reproductive period have had relatively equal chances of giving birth. The relatively uniform fertility structure of these groups requires explanation.

The seven social groups in question do not have similar modes of subsistence. The Bekaa Bedouin and Delta Fulbe of Mali are agropastoralists, the Turkana herders of northern Kenya are pastoralists, the Ganj of Papua New Guinea are horticulturalists, the Ju/'hoansi of Botswana and Namibia are gatherer-hunters, and the Ache of Paraguay and Aka Pygmies of the Central African Republic are hunter-gatherers. It is also evident that these groups do not share a common cultural origin; they are not sister cultures. What can be said is that these groups are politically egalitarian, marginal, small-scale nomadic or seminomadic communities organized along lines of kinship into bands or tribes. Even if we choose not to consider shifting horticulturalists nomadic, the groups in question still share a sociopolitical organization. Social stratification or social categories that designate status groupings are absent. In particular, the Ju/'hoansi,[65] Aka Pygmies,[66] the Ache,[67] the Ganj,[68] and the Bekaa Bedouin have all been described as relatively egalitarian by anthropologists. In Bedouin society, while occupational or economic distinctions are discernable (and could be potential social precursors of class), they have not, at least at this historical juncture, translated into socially designated status hierarchies or hierarchical differences in possession of honor.

Nancy Howell is the first person (of whom I am aware) to draw attention to the Poisson distribution of fertility. Howell observed that the variance in the parity distribution of Ju/'hoansi women is a good fit to the Poisson distribution, and suggests that this may be a distinctive or unique feature of the Ju/'hoansi population.[69] James Wood, Patricia Johnson, and Kenneth Campbell found a similar Poisson pattern among Ganj women.[70] The authors assert that a high degree of uniformity in fertility among women is not unusual or unexpected, given the age pattern of marital fertility observed in other natural-fertility populations provided by Coale and Trussell.[71] Wood, drawing on the Coale-Trussell model fertility schedules, suggests that intra-population fertility differences in natural-fertility populations may be due to more physiological or biological mechanisms (i.e., those less culturally malleable) such as age-related changes in the capacity to conceive and rates of fetal loss.[72] Wood's assertion is basically a description of variation over the female reproductive span; it is a statement about ontogenetic variation. In other words, he is basically stating that, aside from the invariant or incontrovertible biological process of reproductive aging, individual women within a population are relatively homogeneous. The underlying premise is that, within natural fertility populations, women's fertility varies according to age, but little else. While age is clearly one of the most, if not the most, important source of variation among women, there are other sources of local variation (see below).

Poisson distributions are not an invariant feature of natural-fertility populations. Examples of alternative family-size distributions can be found among Herero pastoralists of Ngamiland, Botswana,[73] nomadic Efe foragers, and Lese slash-and-burn farmers of the Democratic Republic of Congo.[74] All three groups have a negative binomial distribution, which can be attributed to the high incidence of sterility associated with the African infertility belt. In other words, high rates of infertility are responsible for the greater heterogeneity in fertility among women in these societies. If the cases of infertility are removed, the distributions would follow a Poisson pattern. Given empirical examples of Poisson distributions in several nomadic, small-scale populations, it is not possible to dismiss reproductive homogeneity as some anomalous or unique feature of a small population or as the result of sampling error. A review of fertility in pretransitional Europe similarly shows that social class or occupational distinctions in fertility at the local level are minimal (see chapter 7).

A Poisson pattern is thus consistent with previous research on women's fertility in European agrarian villages prior to transition. Historical demographic evidence suggests that there is greater variation in mortality than fertility prior to transition.[75] In pointing out the high degree of reproductive homogeneity among women in pretransitional societies worldwide, we must bear in mind that there are taken-for-granted institutionalized practices of marriage, breastfeeding, and so forth, which provide important guidelines for action that individual women draw upon in their reproductive lives. Those same structures, however, always leave room for a diversity of contestations that give rise to social differentiation in fertility as discussed below.

Even though differences in fertility among women within egalitarian societies may be minimal, that does not mean that variation is absent. There is always variation. How do we account for fertility variation within nomadic societies prior to transition? The proximate determinants of fertility are a useful starting point for examining reproductive variation. However, they provide only a partial theory of fertility. The utility of the proximate-determinants framework for anthropological demography and biodemography lies in the recognition that childbearing is a causally complex process that requires attention to both proximate mechanisms, or the "hows" of reproduction, and broader social processes/constraints, or the "whys" of reproduction. Examination of the proximate determinants is not intended to be reductionistic,[76] but to provide more complete hierarchical explanations for reproduction. A hierarchical or scalar approach is grounded in the premise that understanding demographic health variation requires understanding broader socioeconomic structures and underlying biological and social mechanisms contributing to health causation in specific times and places.

In applying the proximate-determinants-of-fertility framework to understand intrapopulation reproductive variation (within nomadic groups), sterility and the age pattern of marriage emerge as important determinants of variation.[77] Primary and secondary sterility help account for much of the intrapopulation variation in fertility worldwide. Howell's examination of the fertility performance of sixty-two Ju/'hoansi women aged forty-five years and older in 1968 revealed that as many as 32 percent of sample women had parity distributions lower than 4. The mean parity and total fertility rate was 4.691.[78] It has been established that the causes of low fertility among

Ju/'hoansi women are pathological sterility due to gonorrhea and other sexually transmitted diseases. Similarly, Pennington and Harpending measured fertility among the Herero of northwestern Botswana, and found that 15 percent of women had no births. The mean parity of 239 postreproductive Herero women in 1986 was 3.47.[79] The authors attribute such low fertility to sterilizing diseases (such as gonorrhea and chlamydia) characteristic of the "African infertility belt," which stretches across central Africa from Tanzania in the east to Gabon in the west.[80] The broader-level force that appears to have produced this pattern of infertility among the Herero is the German genocidal war on the Herero, which occurred between 1904 and 1907.[81]

In contrast, Ache foragers have low rates of sterility and high fertility. At the proximate level, age at first birth is a strong determinant of local variation in Ache fertility.[82] Among Bedouin agropastoralists, who represent another high-fertility and low-sterility population, age at marriage is not a significant determinant of total live births, but marital disruption is (see chapter 4). Bedouin women who experienced widowhood had significantly lower fertility than women who remained continuously in marriage.[83] In examining the parity distributions of 102 postreproductive Bedouin women (see table 2.2), I found that only 6.8 percent of women had completed family sizes of 4 and under. Low fertility can be partially attributed to the failure to remarry when a woman is widowed. Results show that marital stability does not increase fertility; rather, widowhood decreased it. Low fertility is not as prevalent as high fertility among the Bedouin. Approximately 25.5 percent of postreproductive Bedouin women in my sample had completed family sizes greater than 10. The mean parity and total fertility rate was 9.1. One of the women in the group was nulliparous; however, secondary sterility[84] linked to polygynous marriage is a significant predictor of completed family size among women within Bedouin society.

Local variation in fertility needs to be placed in broader historical and political-economic context, or what Andrew Vayda refers to as "progressive contextualization."[85] The high overall rate of sterility in central Africa is ultimately a legacy of colonialism. Most of the proximate causes of intrapopulation variation in egalitarian nomadic societies appear to be sterility and the timing and duration of marriage. However, collectivities of class, ethnicity, race, nationality, and religion may still be relevant to explaining the patterning of fertility and mortality at different scales. If we focus on fertility levels through time, there is some evidence of rising fertility within nomadic communities as a result of greater involvement in agriculture and sedentism.[86] Reduced levels of sterility may also have played a role in rising fertility levels in neocolonial contexts. As mentioned above, low fertility across Africa and the Pacific in the twentieth century is best explained by the effects of STDs. When left untreated, diseases like gonorrhea and chlamydia can lead to pelvic inflammatory disease, which causes permanent damage to the reproductive organs. The "distal," or ultimate, cause of pathologically low fertility in these cases is colonial violence. The most plausible explanation for declining sterility and rising fertility across Africa in the later twentieth century is increased state integration and control, which comes with access to medicines, particularly antibiotics and medical-care facilities.[87] However, we must be careful and not assume that all or most cases of low fertility among foragers or other subsistence groups can be attributed to infectious infertility. For example, low fertility among Ganj swidden horticulturalists in highland New Guinea (4.3 live births per woman) is largely due to breastfeeding/spacing patterns, late menarche and late marriage, and a long interval of over four years between marriage and first birth.[88] Fertility regulation practices in small-scale societies point to the existence of preventive checks that mirror those found in pretransitional societies worldwide (see chapter 6).

Conclusion

A variety of ethnographic studies among nomadic societies from different parts of the world point to the same general conclusion: sociopolitical egalitarianism is not a myth or figment of the romantic anthropological imagination. Ethnographic research among Middle Eastern and African pastoralists has contributed to our understanding of what makes egalitarian societies egalitarian and underscores the necessity of embedding discussions of equality and hierarchy in the continuing history of nomadic peoples—a history often marked by struggle and adjustment to state coercion, colonialism, colonial slavery, and capital accumulation. A review of demographic studies in nomadic societies shows that several groups have been able to maintain local health equity through traditions of food sharing and reciprocity, mobility, and other social means of minimizing or leveling material disparities. A closer look at women's fertility in pastoralist, foraging, and horticultural societies from the Middle East, Africa, Central America, and Oceania similarly reveals that social differentials in fertility are minimal at the local level. Women show a high degree of social integration in their completed family sizes, which is congruent with pretransitional fertility research from Europe discussed in chapter 7. Class hierarchies and class-specific mortality differentials are not universal, but spatially and historically contingent. Social and demographic inequalities at one scale do not necessarily translate into inequalities at another. While it is hard to pin down the hows and whys of egalitarianism, there are forces operating from above—related to political geography and history—and forces operating from below, as individual agents produce and reproduce egalitarian practices and institutions. Egalitarianism is constituted in the dialectic of structure and agency.

9

Conclusions

The North-South demographic divide expresses the global fault line between rich and poor. Roughly one in four people—20 percent of the world's
population—live under extreme poverty.[1] Patterns of morbidity and mortality offer further testimonial to the rift between rich and poor. According to estimates corresponding to the study period, less than 2.5 percent of
the population in rich countries suffer from undernourishment. In poor
countries classified as "less developed," 18 percent of the population is undernourished; this figure rises to 35 percent in "least developed" countries.
The gap in life expectancy between the richest, or "more developed," versus
the poorest, or "least developed," countries is high, at twenty-two years. The
average life expectancy at birth is seventy-seven years for "more developed"
countries, sixty-seven years for "less developed" countries including China,
sixty-five years for "less developed" countries excluding China, and fifty-five
years for the "least developed" countries. Much of the gap in life expectancy
is attributable to differentials in infant mortality. Infant mortality in "more
developed" countries is estimated at six infant deaths per one thousand
births; in the "least developed" countries, it is estimated at eighty-five infant
deaths per one thousand births. The region with the lowest infant-mortality
rates in the world is Europe, while sub-Saharan Africa has the highest rates.[2]

The global fertility divide between rich and poor has narrowed, but is
still visible. Women now average 2.6 children during their lifetimes, 3.2 in
"developing countries" excluding China, and 4.7 in the "least developed"
countries. Relatively higher fertility remains in sub-Saharan Africa and the
Middle Eastern countries of Yemen (TFR = 6.2), Afghanistan (TFR = 6.8),
Iraq (TFR = 4.6), and Pakistan (TFR = 4.0).[3] Pockets of high fertility are
also found among smaller social groups, including Bedouin communities
living within or between the borders of nation-states in the Middle East.
In spite of the overall decline in total fertility rates in poor countries, these
countries will still experience rapid population growth due to population
momentum, while wealthy countries will experience little growth and even

decline. Roughly 17.9 percent of the world's population live in countries classified as rich, while 82.1 percent of people in the world reside in poor countries—those designated as "less developed" and "least developed." The share of the world's population living in poorer countries has increased dramatically over the last half century. In 1950, when the population of the world was 2.5 billion, 68 percent of the world's population were living in Africa, Asia, Latin America, and the Caribbean, compared to 82 percent in 2008. The rich countries are projected to lose an additional 4 percent of their 18 percent share of the world's population by 2050.[4]

Global geographic disparities in the demographic profiles of rich and poor invoke political cleavages of colonizer-colonized and center-periphery in the modern capitalist system.[5] Karl Marx wrote about the relationship between capital, labor, and population, particularly the tendency of capital to increase the industrial population, or labor pool. Above all, his work recognized how classes on one side of the capitalist system accumulate capital by exploitation or by appropriating for themselves not simply the resources but the surplus labor of those on the other side of the capitalist divide. As a result, one side accumulates "wealth," while the other side accumulates "misery."[6] Behind the Manichaean structure of the world demographic landscape lies a dismal truth—one that suggests that not all of the familiar binaries of interpretation are to be rejected. On a global level and at some other scales, social polarities point to exploitative political economies—the transference of value from periphery to center. But we should not be surprised to learn that the measure and meaning of demographic differences do not always conform to the conjectures of class. To universalize dichotomies of class, race, and gender without attention to time-space conditions is to miss the variegations of power and resistance and to posit social laws akin to natural ones—in effect, naturalizing power in human societies.

One aim in writing this book has been to situate Bedouin reproductive behavior in political-economic context that is sensitive to both geography and history. The picture of demographic differentiation that is painted is admittedly complex, but it is a complexity that is accessible and points to the utility of a critical political-economy framework. As I have attempted to show in the book, there is a high degree of social and demographic equality within Bekaa Bedouin society and other egalitarian communities that rely on kinship ties, sharing, and reciprocity. Very high Bedouin fertility is historically found in conjunction with moderate overall mortality, high nutritional status, minor gender disparities in child survival, and an overall lack of classlike or occupational disparities in health. Class relations and class-specific demographic differentials are apparent at different scales—

between Bedouin and peasant groups in the Bekaa region, with Bedouin having higher fertility and mortality—prompting us to pay closer attention to the contingencies of geography and history when examining rich/poor divides. I have argued that class distinctions between Bedouins and peasants and the fertility and mortality distinctions accompanying them are linked to a host of changes, most notably the revolution in transport and industrial production of animal feed, which initiated a more sedentary agrarian way of life among the Bedouin. As Bedouin families gradually sold off livestock to purchase land on which to build permanent homes, they became increasingly alienated from their herds. Through "progressive contextualization," local transformations can be connected to broader political-economic processes.

Bedouin fertility decline occurred years after that of proletarianized and landed peasants in the Bekaa Valley and several decades after that of more urbanized segments of Lebanon's overall population. A comparison of fertility between similar age cohorts of Bedouin and non-Bedouin Arab women in the Bekaa shows pronounced differentials, with Bedouin women having higher fertility. Infant- and child-mortality rates also differ between the social groups, with Bedouin children suffering higher mortality. Fertility regulation was not unknown among older Bedouin women who used withdrawal and breastfeeding for spacing and late stopping. Fertility estimates among postreproductive Bedouin women show that Bedouin fertility is high by world standards and constitutes one of the highest fertility rates ever recorded, at approximately nine births per woman. The overall level of infant and child mortality in Bekaa Bedouin society is higher than that found in the general population in Lebanon, but is still moderate compared to that found in marginalized agropastoral groups worldwide. Likewise, Bedouin life expectancy is on par with the global average (for the year 2000), and Bedouin nutritional status points to dietary adequacy. Contrary to Malthusian assumptions, very high fertility does not necessarily precipitate death, disease, and pauperism. Neither is very high fertility an invariant feature of Bedouin society, but is confined to a particular historical period.

Historical estimates indicate that Bedouin completed fertility was high, at 6.8 live births, but not very high, during the beginning decades of the twentieth century. Fertility increased among cohorts of women born during the late French Mandate years and independence period. These women were marrying and beginning their childbearing between the 1960s and 1980s—a period of major economic transition, in which Bedouins were establishing villages and increasingly turning to farming and wage labor, as well as industrial feed for livestock-rearing (which may have raised the Malthusian population ceiling for Bedouin). Over the long term, changes accompanying modernization eventually precipitated a decline in Bedouin fertility—the total-period fertility rate in 2000 is estimated at 6.55. As Bedouin became alienated from their herds and traditional grazing lands, they were left with their labor power to sell or exchange for a share of the harvest in sharecropping contracts. Bedouin fertility decline coincides with a downward trend in the Lebanese economy, particularly galloping inflation beginning in the mid-1980s, which raised the cost of living. The economic strain of maintaining a large family in a consumer capitalist society is increasingly felt by Bedouin families. Fertility was high when consumption was low. High fertility did not induce a Malthusian catastrophe, because Bedouin consumed little, reaped the benefits of family labor, and enjoyed the security provided by the keeping of livestock in a mixed economy. Newly married Bedouin couples interviewed in 2007 appear to be adjusting their fertility goals to meet their new economic circumstances. Bedouin women are increasingly receptive to using modern contraception (IUD and the pill) to control their fertility within marriage. Younger couples express a desire for smaller families, which mothers and fathers say are necessary if they are to provide their children with appropriate food, clothing, and education. The challenges facing Bedouin today are common among peoples who have experienced capitalist dispossession, proletarianization, and state regulation. It is precisely these new economic circumstances that threaten to undermine future Bedouin health, as previously interdependent economic relations with peasants have given way to more exploitative ones based on manifestly unequal access to the means of production and political power.

The distinct profiles of birth and death and the distinct timing of transition between Bedouin and peasant groups in the Bekaa Valley, Lebanon, point to a differential demography of classes akin to those documented in anthropological demographic studies from Europe. However, it is difficult to draw similar inferences about economic inequality within Bedouin communities. Economic wealth and occupation exert minimal influence on both the number of Bedouin children ever born and the number of surviving children. Birth spacing, marital disruption (due to widowhood), and subfertility on the part of polygynous first wives account for most of the internal variation in Bedouin fertility. Infant and child mortality are more responsive to birth interval length, birth order, and consanguinity than economic inequities. Even in Europe, demographic variegations are more common than is generally acknowledged. If we look at the unfolding of demographic inequities in time and their distribution in space, there appears to be little empirical support for class differences in fertility between women at local levels in Europe prior to transition. In contrast, pretransitional class or occupational differentials in early mortality and life expectancy are discernable, but here too mortality shows variations contingent on local institutional practices of breastfeeding and child care.

The moderate overall level of Bedouin mortality signals that the epidemiological transition is under way. The absence of occupational differentials in infant and child deaths in Bedouin communities points to incongruities in the social configurations of class in time and place. Through food-sharing, hospitality, rules prohibiting the sale of labor to others within the community, humor, and other checks to power, nomadic peoples have upheld egalitarian practices and warded off potential status distinctions of wealth, tribe, and the like. Mobility itself is an important means by which nomadic peoples resist state power, escape colonial military aggression,[7] evade tax collection, and avoid wealth accumulation. (The modern political delineation of national territories has made mobility for nomadic peoples more difficult.) Implicated in egalitarian practices are specific sociohistorical and geographical conditions, expressly the intersocietal system of conjunctive relations between nomads and the state. In peripheral areas where state power was weak (or weakened by fighting between states), nomads were organized into smaller and less hierarchical groups. Concepts like "peripheral," "remote," and "isolated" are not ecological givens but direct attention to political-geographic realities of encapsulation/autonomy.

Nomadic societies are not alone in offsetting social hierarchies through horizontal ties. Historical demographic research from Europe shows how shared patterns of breastfeeding cut across class lines to keep infant mortality low in several localities. Some contemporary socialist democracies are able to level off economic inequalities in health by offering adequate unemployment protections and other social safety nets (at least for state citizens, if not for noncitizens). In countries like the United States that lack these safety nets, adverse health effects of income inequities are more pronounced.[8]

Kinship is believed to be an important social means of circumventing vertical hierarchies of class in human societies. Yet kinship-centered practices like consanguineous marriage are not inherently anticlass. Class cleavages can potentially be reinforced by encouraging marriage between kin of a particular social class. In Bedouin communities of the Bekaa Valley, wage laborers are less likely to marry their first cousins than pastoralists and sharecroppers, but still marry within their tribe. The broader shared tribal affiliation of couples cuts across socioeconomic distinctions, implying that the communal links of tribal organization overshadow asymmetries of occupation. Kinship norms surrounding marriage must continuously be interpreted and acted upon by human agents who differ in their interests and positionality. This means that normative structures are open to transformation and interpolation. By marrying relatives, individuals reproduce social kinship structures. The cultural preference for marriage between a man and his father's brother's daughter (patriparallel cousin) would be incongruous if the patrilineal society in question automatically bestowed full kinship to a man's descendants irrespective of his wife. It is the woman's consanguineous relationship with her spouse that determines authentic kinship. Kinship rests on the attribution of specific identities to other persons, which, in turn, intersects with identities of gender and occupation. Bedouin women who marry within their parental camp can also draw upon the face-to-face support of family members to check the husband's authority.

The demographic and family lives of Arabs are construed far differently under the yoke of colonialism and imperialism. Marriage and procreation are viewed less as expressions of personhood and more as products of a domineering male culture. Euramerican stereotypes of Arab societies as repositories of culturally backward and oppressive traditions that victimize women help invite and validate colonialism. Cultural inferiority fills in for racial inferiority, but does not entirely replace the latter. Eugenic concerns over the racial makeup of a population have been reignited in the wake of the second demographic transition. As fertility drops and stays well below replacement level in post-transitional metropolitan countries, the shrinking and rapid aging of populations are expected, making the replacement of future generations difficult, unless migration compensates for the demographic imbalance. In this context, low white fertility and high nonwhite fertility are imbued with added significance.

During the last several decades, the concept of "culture" has come under serious anthropological scrutiny over its complicity with power. James Clifford's *The Predicament of Culture* details the essentialist, static, and reified narratives of culture.[9] In the wake of the latter, Abu-Lughod's "Writing against Culture"[10] has picked up momentum as anthropologists from different subfields have identified similar theoretical and political problems with culture: culture "asked to do the work of race,"[11] the tendency of scholars "to confuse structural violence with cultural difference,"[12] and culture and "culture talk" reflecting a failure of political-historical analysis and colonial attempts to justify the use of military force.[13] Of particular importance for anthropologists working across subfields is to elucidate how inequities of power, under the aegis of culture, serve to re-create both classism and racism. While I believe that there are elements of the culture concept worth retaining, the concept of the "duality of structure" impels us to recognize that culture can be garnered to either destabilize or validate imperial power.[14] Culture is never immutable. Meaning, norms, and power are fluid in their applications and open to contestation.

Representations of gender—intimately linked to culture and power— also risk turning the concept into a monolithic category. If we recognize that the concept of woman operates through a conjunction of interlocking structures of class, race, and the like, then we are less inclined to accept that the experiences of oppression endured by one group of women (white middle-class women) can sufficiently capture the struggles of other women. By separating gender from race and class, we are left with an abstract and universalistic concept of gender that naturalizes and thus negates itself.

Unfavorable colonial constructions of Arab culture and gender turn the focus away from the colonizer and toward the colonized. By portraying colonized peoples as "inferior," "brutish," "backward," and in need of "emancipation," the colonizer blame-shifts and redefines acts of colonization. Ironically, postcolonial subjects in the Middle East today, vis-à-vis sentiments toward Bedouin tribal peoples, mimic and reinforce the colonial epithetization of primitives. (Favorable Rousseauian imagery that creates a fixed view of Bedouin as relics of an imagined past who pose no serious threat to power, owing to their minority status and limited access to the means of coercion, is more of an exception that proves the rule.) The (c)overt violence lurking behind modern, colonialist constructions of Arab-Muslim peoples is thinly disguised. Arab-Muslim societies have been subject to both discursive and military attack. Like the oxymoronic "noble savage," the Muslim who cooperates with colonial power is exalted as "good," and s/he who does not is decried as "bad." It is the logic of violent racial imperialism: might makes right and white makes right. Mexican philosopher Enrique Dussel argues that the violent heritage of modernity can be traced to the expansion of Europe over the last five hundred years.[15] Like the corporal punishment of children that's said to be "for their own good," the violent assimilation and subordination of "savages" is believed to be the cost of developmental civilizational progress. Death and human suffering are merely the "growing pains" of civilization. Conventional narratives of Arab reproduction similarly rest on denigrations of Arab men, the Arab family, and the so-called agentless Arab woman-victim. High fertility, consanguineous marriage, and polygyny are seen as Oriental, demographic maladies that demand an Occidental cure.

The study of demography and health has the potential to broaden our understanding of structures of power and domination. Efforts to discuss women's freedom and reproductive liberty without addressing colonialism, racial imperialism, and capitalism[16] are bound to be incomplete. The modern-day embrace of low-fertility norms and practices is based in part on the classist and racist juxtaposition of large poor families (linked to the rural poor in the global South) against small prosperous families (linked to elite classes in the global North and South)—with the latter serving as the superior social ideal. Such a view not only stigmatizes poor people of color and poor whites who do not live up to white bourgeois fertility norms, but fails to acknowledge the existence of alternative demographic regimes in which health, liberty, and economic well-being are not contingent upon low fertility.

Because steady fertility declines have occurred in the metropole and most regions of the global South, without a parallel global decrease in the economic gap between rich and poor, we are in a position to reject the Malthusian inference that small nuclear families built around individualism will usher in a golden age of economic prosperity. As critical interlocutors of power, we can also identify in Malthusian/neo-Malthusian theory the colonial chastisement of poor women of color and their reproductive capacity. Both then and now, much of what the colonizer fears and therefore disparages is the demographic power in numbers—an industrial reserve army turned reserve army that outmuscles or outreproduces the other side.

The convergence of colonialism and social justice motivates us to seek a liberation that negates the tenets of imperialism and embraces non-Eurocentric alterity. The endeavors of the "liberal," "democratic," capitalist state and its agencies to colonize peoples with one hand and promise "freedom" with the other should by now be familiar colonial hoaxes. For these reasons, we would do well to explore concepts of justice outside of the context of reproductive control and state-authorized "human rights" discourse. A colonial and imperial liberalism that remonstrates against inequities of race, class, and gender while, at the same time, bending to the needs of capital and the military patriarchal state only re-creates a world in its own fractured image.

Notes

Chapter 1. Introduction and Overview

1. Kent and Haub, "Global Demographic Divide," 3.

2. See Sen, "Population: Delusion and Reality"; Laughlin, "Evolution of Modern Demography"; and Hartmann, *Reproductive Rights and Wrongs*.

3. Giddens, *Transformation of Intimacy*, 26.

4. Ibid., 27.

5. Laughlin, "Evolution of Modern Demography."

6. See, for instance, Scheper-Hughes, *Death without Weeping*; Ali, *Planning the Family in Egypt*; Van Hollen, *Birth on the Threshold*; Thomas, *Politics of the Womb*; Maternowska, *Reproducing Inequities*; Fadlalla, *Embodying Honor*; Briggs, *Reproducing Empire*; Bledsoe, *Contingent Lives*; Kanaaneh, *Birthing the Nation*; Johnson-Hanks, *Uncertain Honor*; and Rivkin-Fish, *Women's Health in Post-Soviet Russia*.

7. See, for instance, Caldwell, Reddy, and Caldwell, *Causes of Demographic Change*; Das Gupta, "Fertility Decline in Punjab, India"; Fricke, *Himalayan Households*; Greenhalgh, "Fertility as Mobility"; Greenhalgh, "Controlling Births and Bodies"; Greenhalgh, "Anthropology Theorizes Reproduction"; Kertzer and Hogan, *Demographic Change*; Lockwood, *Fertility and Household Labour*; Schneider and Schneider, *Festival of the Poor*; Netting, *Balancing on an Alp*; Renne, "Nigerian Land Use" and *Population and Progress*; and Weinreb, "First Politics, Then Culture."

8. See, for instance, Howell, *Demography of the Dobe !Kung*; Wood, *Dynamics of Human Reproduction*; Hill and Hurtado, *Ache Life History*; Pennington and Harpending, *African Pastoralist Community*; Chamberlain, *Demography in Archaeology*; Early and Headland, *Population Dynamics*; Early and Peters, *Xilixana Yanomami of the Amazon*; Panter-Brick, Layton, and Rowley-Conwy, *Hunter-Gatherers*; and Blurton Jones et al., "Demography of the Hadza."

9. See, for instance, Borgerhoff Mulder, "Datoga Pastoralists of Tanzania"; Borgerhoff Mulder and Sellen, "Pastoralist Decision-Making"; Fratkin, Galvin, and Roth, *African Pastoralist Systems*; and Roth, "On Pastoralist Egalitarianism."

10. See Joseph, "Biocultural Context"; Joseph, "Globalization, Demography and Nutrition"; and Joseph, "'Kissing Cousins.'"

11. See Bittles, "Consanguinity as a Demographic Variable"; and Bittles, "Consanguinity and Its Relevance."

12. Fischer, *Historians' Fallacies*, 5.

13. Malthus, *Principle of Population*, 14–15.

14. Ibid., 57.

15. Farmer, "An Anthropology of Structural Violence."

16. Borofsky, "Four Subfields," 464.

17. Goodman and Leatherman, *Building a New Biocultural Synthesis*.

18. See Baer, Singer, and Susser, *Medical Anthropology*.

19. See Guess, *Critical Theory*.

20. In a landmark volume by David Kertzer and Tom Fricke, *Anthropological Demography*, contributors attempted to lay out a vision for the liaison between anthropology and demography, but this synthesis almost entirely excluded the contributions of biodemography. An important exception is Eric Roth's *Culture, Biology and Anthropological Demography*, which has attempted to reconcile anthropological demography and evolutionary ecology. A public health focus has always characterized the field. The aforementioned (landmark) edited volume and another edited compilation in the same field by Alaka Basu and Peter Aaby entitled *The Methods and Uses of Anthropological Demography* are testimonies to that.

21. Konner, *Tangled Wing*, 496.

22. See Habermas, *Between Facts and Norms*.

23. See Greenhalgh "Toward a Political Economy." See also Habermas, *Between Facts and Norms*.

24. Macey, *Penguin Dictionary of Critical Theory*, 75 (italics in the original).

25. Spivak, "Righting Wrongs," 524.

26. Hartmann, *Reproductive Rights and Wrongs*, 116. See also Connelly, *Fatal Mis-Conception*.

27. Connelly, *Fatal Mis-Conception*, 382.

28. Ibid., 374.

29. Ibid., 381.

30. I use the term "Fourth World" to refer to semi/nomadic pastoral, foraging, and horticultural communities as well as indigenous peoples marginalized from the dominant culture. The term may also be used to refer to what Geertz refers to as the "exprimitive." Geertz, "Devastation of the Amazon," 133.

31. bell hooks, *Ain't I a Woman*, 190.

32. Kraft, "Hunt for Genes."

33. Ibid.

34. Visweswaran, "Race."

35. See Said, *Orientalism*. This Orientalist perspective has even been internalized by Arab writers themselves (see Massad, *Desiring Arabs*).

36. Paul, "Orientalism Revisited," 47.

37. See Freedman et al., "Life History Calendar."

38. Minor corrections were made to original age estimates, which resulted in a one-year age adjustment for five women in my sample.

39. See Howell, *Demography of the Dobe !Kung*.

40. All anthropometric measurements were taken following the protocols of Lohman, Roache, and Martorell, *Anthropometric Standardization Reference Manual*.

41. For a description of the method used to derive a wealth index of the basic means of production, see Sheridan, *Where the Dove Calls*.

42. See El-Kholy and Al-Ali, "Inside/Out."

43. Chatty, "Bedouin in Lebanon."

44. National-level estimates place total financial losses in livestock production due to the war at US$21,861,845. FAO Technical Cooperation Programme, *Lebanon*, 17.

Chapter 2. Nomadic Lives in Transition

1. Cultural anthropologist Dawn Chatty has described traditional Bedouin nomadism and the transition to modern sedentary life in some detail in her dissertation (conducted in the Bekaa between 1972 and 1973), which was published as a monograph, in 1986, entitled *From Camel to Truck: The Bedouin in the Modern World*. Fadl Al-Faour, a Bedouin shaykh, completed the first dissertation on the Bedouin in the Bekaa region in 1968. The ethnographic research for his dissertation—which is entitled "Social Structure of a Bedouin Tribe in the Syria-Lebanon Region"—was carried out between 1962 and 1963.

2. Chatty, "From Camel to Truck: A Study of the Pastoral Economy of the Al-Fadl and Al-Hassana in the Bekaa Valley, Lebanon."

3. The Bekaa continues to comprise about 68 percent of the total number of sheep (279,000), 44 percent of goats (206,000), and 28 percent of cows (22,000) in the country. Lebanon Ministry of Agriculture, *National Action Programme to Combat Desertification*, 72. For information on the distribution of livestock and agricultural holdings in the Bekaa, see chapter 3.

4. Chatty, "Bedouin in Lebanon."

5. Lebanon Ministry of Agriculture, *National Action Programme to Combat Desertification*, 70.

6. Lebanon Ministry of Agriculture, *Agricultural Statistics Lebanon 2005*, 10.

7. Velud, "French Mandate Policy."

8. Ibid.

9. Chatty, "Bedouin in Lebanon."

10. Chatty, "From Camel to Truck: A Study of the Pastoral Economy of the Al-Fadl and Al-Hassana in the Bekaa Valley, Lebanon," 111.

11. I also obtained parental occupation for 216 of the women's spouses, but these are not presented.

12. Wood, "Fertility in Anthropological Populations."

13. Campbell and Wood, "Fertility in Traditional Societies."

14. Harpending and Draper, "Estimating Parity of Parents."

15. Ibid.

16. See note 13 above.

17. Eltigani, "Fertility Transition in Arab Countries," 169.

18. Ibid., 164. During the same period, Asia and Oceania experienced a 29 percent decline, Latin America and the Caribbean 15 percent, and sub-Saharan Africa 17 percent (ibid.).

19. Lebanon Ministry of Agriculture, *National Action Programme to Combat Desertification*, 79. This population estimate for the Bekaa is from 1997, which roughly coincides with the time of my fieldwork in 2000.

20. El Kak, "Bedouin Health Provision."

21. Chatty, "Bedouin in Lebanon."

22. Ibid., 26. The political structure of Lebanon as established in the 1943 National Pact allocates power on a confessional system based on the 1932 census and its findings of a slight Christian majority in Lebanon. The confessional system guarantees Christian political domination in Lebanon. The president is to be a Maronite Christian, the speaker of the parliament a Shi'i Muslim, and the prime minister a Sunni Muslim. Twelve seats in parliament were divided on a 6-to-5 ratio of Christians to Muslims until a balanced ratio replaced it in 1990. Because Christians no longer represent a majority in Lebanon, Christian Lebanese authorities have been reluctant to undertake a population census.

23. Held and Cummings, *Middle East Patterns,* 294.

24. "WFP Starts Distributing Food Vouchers."

25. Lebanon Ministry of Agriculture, *National Action Programme to Combat Desertification*, 79, table 3.1.

26. See Daher, *Socio-Economic Changes*, 44–45, 50.

27. Lebanon Ministry of Agriculture, *National Action Programme to Combat Desertification*.

28. Lebanon Ministry of Agriculture, *Agricultural Statistics Lebanon 2005*, 10, table 6. In comparison, the distribution of the country's harvested crop area—both rain-fed and irrigated production—consisted of fruit trees (28 percent), cereals (24 percent), olives (22 percent), vegetables (15 percent), agro-industrial crops (4 percent), legumes (3 percent), other trees (2%), and other crops (2 percent) (ibid.).

29. Lebanon Ministry of Agriculture, *National Action Programme to Combat Desertification*, 79.

30. See FAO Technical Cooperation Programme, *Lebanon*.

31. Held and Cummings, *Middle East Patterns*, 301–2.

32. Ratha and Xu, *Migration and Remittances Factbook 2008*, 17. See also Ghosh, *Migrants' Remittances and Development*; and Gebara, *Reconstruction Survey*.

33. See note 26 above.

34. Held and Cummings, *Middle East Patterns*, 292.

35. Daher, *Socio-Economic Changes*, 44.

36. Issawi, *Economic History*; and Daher, *Socio-Economic Changes*, 51.

37. See Gebara, *Reconstruction Survey*.

38. Laithy, Abu-Ismail, and Hamdan, "Poverty, Growth and Income Distribution."

39. Lebanon Ministry of Agriculture, *National Action Programme to Combat Desertification*, 83. Estimates of the average annual income of a Lebanese family vary, but one

estimate put it at US$12,000 in 2001. Center for Research on Population and Health, *Patterns of Household Income*.

40. Saidi, *War in Lebanon*; Lebanon Ministry of Agriculture, *National Action Programme to Combat Desertification*; and Daher, *Socio-Economic Changes*.

41. Daher, *Socio-Economic Changes*, 107.

Chapter 3. (Un)Stratified Reproduction

1. See Braveman and Tarimo, "Social Inequalities"; Marmot, "Achieving Health Equity"; and Sastry, "Trends in Socioeconomic Inequalities"; and CSDH, *Closing the Gap*.

2. Colen, "'Like a Mother to Them.'"

3. One Bedouin woman married to her ibn 'amm [patriparallel cousin] referred to the tattoo on her forearm as "the pillow of my ibn 'amm." Her cousin-spouse was supposed to rest his head on her tattooed arm. As she was explaining the meaning behind her tattoo, her sister-in-law (i.e., husband's brother's wife) interjected by teasing that the husband in question was often denied the comforts of "his pillow." The woman's marriage to her ibn 'amm was one of the few forced marriages I encountered.

4. Patron-client relations are based on differential power and authority. Patron-client ties are present between peasant landowning families and Bedouins who work the land as sharecroppers and between Lebanese landowners and the Bedouin families who graze their flocks on peasant fields year after year. Pastoralists allow their daughters to perform agricultural labor for peasant landowners in return for permission to graze on their land. Bedouin will sometimes approach a landowner if they need to borrow money to cover work or medical expenses or, in one instance I observed, to purchase prescription eyeglasses for a child.

5. Thomas Barfield (*Nomadic Alternative*, 74) explains how Bedouin hospitality is historically tied to the desert environment in which Bedouins lived. Reciprocal obligations of hospitality help make travel and survival in the desert possible, especially in areas where tents are few and towns are far. Middle Eastern nomads in Iran and Afghanistan who reside next to villages and towns have a different hospitality ethic from Bedouins. According to Barfield, the former will usually direct unknown visitors to the closest "caravanserai" after a more modest welcome that includes a cup of tea.

6. Daher, *Socio-Economic Changes*.

7. ECODIT and Lebanon Ministry of Environment/LEDO, *State of the Environment Report*.

8. Lebanon Ministry of Agriculture, *National Action Programme to Combat Desertification*, 70.

9. Ibid., 73, table 2.15.

10. Lebanon Ministry of Public Health, *Maternal and Child Health Survey*.

11. Ibid.

12. The infant mortality rate for the total country was estimated at 28 per 1,000 in 1995. "Lebanon 1996," 178.

13. *United Nations Demographic Yearbook, 2000.*

14. Kulczycki and Saxena, "Population, Environment, and Health Nexus."

15. World Health Organization, *World Health Report 2001.*

16. Observatory/EMRO/WHO, *Health System Profile--Lebanon.*

17. "Lebanon 1996," 175.

18. See Lebanon Ministry of Public Health, *Maternal and Child Health Survey,* 7–9. See also "Lebanon 1996."

19. Chatty, "Bedouin in Lebanon."

20. Cole, "Where Have the Bedouin Gone?"

21. Ibid.

22. Kreager, "Demographic Regimes as Cultural Systems," 153–55.

23. Schneider and Schneider, *Festival of the Poor,* 11.

24. See Tamari, "Persistence of Sharetenancy."

25. See Pollock, "Sharecropping."

26. Ibid.

27. Following Kreager ("Demographic Regimes as Cultural Systems"), "demographic regime" is defined as a property of all societies and includes a system of regularities in marriage and the onset of sexual relations, fertility, breastfeeding, relations of age, class, gender, and kinship, child-rearing customs, emigration and immigration, and property transmission. See also Schneider and Schneider, *Festival of the Poor,* 196–97.

28. The unadjusted logistic regression results indicate that wealth (ownership of the basic means of production in livestock, land and machinery) has a *negative* impact on child mortality; however, the unadjusted logistic regression model should be approached with caution, as it does not include appropriate statistical controls. Joseph, "'Kissing Cousins.'"

29. See Bradburd, *Ambiguous Relations;* Laclau, *Politics and Ideology;* and Dupré and Rey, "History of Exchange."

30. Frank et al., "Genes and the Environment."

31. See Bittles, "Consanguinity as a Demographic Variable."

32. Joseph, "'Kissing Cousins.'"

33. The two primary proximate mechanisms by which birth spacing is believed to influence mortality are maternal depletion and sibling competition (Whitworth and Stephenson, "Birth Spacing"). Maternal depletion syndrome refers to the fact that short intervals between births do not allow the mother adequate time to achieve the nutritional status that she has in a nonpregnant, nonlactating state. The child succeeding the short interval is thus at a disadvantage both in terms of fetal malnutrition and a compromised intrauterine environment. Sibling competition or rivalry is the other mechanism by which short intervals increase the mortality risk of infants and young children. In situations where two or more young children close in age are competing for maternal care and attention, this can negatively impact the nutritional status of the index child as well as increase the risk of morbidity/mortality due to illness and accidents. Because Bedouin women have adequate nutrient reserves, it is likely that sibling competition is the primary mechanism by which short preceding birth interval increases the risk of infant and child

mortality. See also Curtis, Diamond, and McDonald, "Birth Interval" and Forste, "Effects of Breastfeeding."

34. See note 32 above.

35. Other demographic studies have reported a similar pattern with regard to birth-order position. See Modin, "Birth Order and Mortality."

36. See note 32 above.

37. National Society of Genetic Counselors, "First Cousins Face Lower Risk."

38. Lebanon Department of Health and Vital Statistics, *Statistical Bulletin 2007*, 33.

39. Ibid., 34.

40. Billig, *Freudian Repression*, 100. Billig argues that repression is better understood in terms of language and culture. Because repression encompasses a diversity of topics that are not fixed in time and place, repression has no universal meaning and cannot be reduced to biological drives of either a sexual or aggressive nature.

41. Lindholm, "Kinship Structure and Political Authority."

42. Evans-Pritchard, *Nuer*.

43. Sahlins, "Segmentary Lineage System."

44. For another example of a brother homicide in the region, see Al-Faour, "Social Structure," 187.

45. As previously mentioned, there were a few reported cases of Syrian Bedouins working as hired shepherds for Lebanese Bedouin families early in the family life cycle when labor is scarce. However, I did not obtain demographic measures of fertility and infant and child mortality from hired Syrian shepherds, as many of these individuals were employed by Lebanese pastoralists before the fieldwork period. Hence, I cannot verify whether or not there are fertility and mortality distinctions between hired Syrian Bedouin shepherds and their Lebanese Bedouin employers.

Chapter 4. Gender Myths and Demographic Realities

1. See Kanaaneh, *Birthing the Nation*.

2. Mainstream feminist groups like the Fund for a Feminist Majority have supported the U.S.-led war in Afghanistan on the pretext that it is a fight to "liberate" Afghan women. Smith, *Conquest*.

3. See Johnson-Hanks, "Muslim Fertility." See also Inhorn and Sargent, "Introduction to Medical Anthropology."

4. Ahmed, *Women and Gender in Islam*.

5. Ibid., 151.

6. Smith, *Conquest*, 23.

7. Gayatri Spivak's expression "white men are saving brown women from brown men" succinctly captures these colonial dissimulations. "Can the Subaltern Speak?" 33.

8. Ahmed, *Women and Gender in Islam*, 151.

9. Winckler, *Arab Political Demography*, 45.

10. Connelly, *Fatal Mis-Conception*, 312.

11. Hartmann, *Reproductive Rights and Wrongs*, 43.

12. Ibid., 48.

13. Ibid.

14. See Mahmood, "Feminist Theory."

15. Benjamin, *Bonds of Love*, 83.

16. Mohanty, "Under Western Eyes," 333.

17. Hoagland defines heterosexualism as a particular type of institutionalized relationship (political, economic, and emotional) between men and women that promotes
the subordination of the latter to the former and prevents the latter from building and
sustaining communities of women. Hoagland, "Heterosexualism and White Supremacy,"
166.

18. Ibid., 168.

19. The female biological advantage is not absolute, but subject to time-space fluc-
tuation depending on sociotechnological and socioecological conditions. Measles is frequently more lethal for girls than boys, since girls tend to be infected by higher-level doses
of the virus found within the more confined spaces of the home (Aaby et al., "Cross-Sex
Transmission"). Studies are needed that look into gender-specific measles mortality and
cross-gender as well as intra-gender measles transmission in Lebanon and other countries
in the region with high measles rates before any firm conclusions can be drawn about the
causes of gender differentials in disease mortality in the Middle East. It is also necessary
to consider the impact that changes in medical technology in the region have had on the
gender gap in early mortality. The male infant-mortality disadvantage in rich countries
has been shrinking since 1970 due to medical technological developments. The spread
of Cesarean delivery and neonatal intensive care units has reduced infant mortality, dis-
proportionately benefiting males since male infants are more likely to be born premature
or with low birth weight, and full-term male infants are more likely to suffer delivery
complications, owing to their larger body size and head circumference (Drevenstedt et
al., "Excess Male Infant Mortality").

20. Hill and Upchurch, "Evidence of Gender Differences."

21. Jordan Department of Statistics and Macro International Inc., *Family Health Survey 1997*.

22. Al-Jaber and Farid, *Qatar Family Health Survey 1998*.

23. Alnesef, Al-Rashoud, and Farid, *Kuwait Family Health Survey 1996*.

24. Fikri and Farid, *United Arab Emirates Family Health Survey 1995*. The demographic composition of the United Arab Emirates is unique in that roughly 80 percent
of the population consists of foreign expats.

25. For a review of demographic data on child health in the Middle East from the
1970s and 1980s, see Yount, "Excess Mortality of Girls," and, from the 1990s, see Khawaja et al., "Disparities in Child Health." There are some historical anomalies. For example, Yount's study reports excess female infant mortality in Jordan during the 1970s
and 1980s, whereas Khawaja et al. report that female infants had an advantage in Jordan
during the 1990s. The same turnaround is found in Algeria with respect to female child
mortality. Excess female one to four mortality in Algeria during the 1970s and 1980s had
shifted to a female advantage in the 1990s.

26. Palestinian refugees constitute an important exception to this pattern. Child mortality is higher than infant mortality in Palestinian refugee camps in Gaza, Lebanon, Jordan, and Syria (Madi, "Palestinian Refugee Populations"). Inadequate public health facilities in the refugee camps—linked to broader political realities of Zionist colonialism, expulsion, and dispossession—are responsible for this unusual mortality pattern.

27. An early-child-mortality pattern distinct from that of other Arab countries was found in Saudi Arabia during the mid-1990s. Infant mortality was higher for females (21.8) than males (21.1) in Saudi Arabia, whereas child mortality was higher for males (9.2) than females (5.1). Nevertheless, under-five mortality was still higher for males (30.1) than females (20.6) (Khoja and Farid, *Saudi Arabia Family Health Survey 1996*, 185).

28. Information on the nutritional and health status of children shows that a greater proportion of male children in Syria are underweight, stunted, and suffer a higher prevalence of diarrhea as well as cough. In addition, a lower proportion of male children in Syria are fully immunized. However, the level of consultation for treatment of diarrhea was slightly higher for male children (65 percent) than female children (63 percent) (Syrian Arab Republic, *Maternal and Child Health Survey*, 8). Likewise, the level of consultation for a cough was higher for male children (83 percent) than for female children (80 percent) in Syria (ibid., 10). Lebanon similarly has a higher prevalence of diarrhea, cough, and accidents among male children, as well as a lower proportion of male children who are fully immunized. The level of consultation for treatment of a cough was higher for boys than girls in Lebanon, although comparative percentages are not provided (Lebanon Ministry of Public Health, *Maternal and Child Health Survey*). See also "Lebanon 1996."

29. Coale and Demeny, *Regional Model Life Tables*.

30. Giddens, *Central Problems in Social Theory* and Giddens, *New Rules of Sociological Method*.

31. Giddens, *Transformation of Intimacy*, 27.

32. Russell, *Power*.

33. Ibid., 8.

34. Giddens, *Central Problems in Social Theory*, 91.

35. Ibid., 100 (italics in the original).

36. Both Shamsa and her senior co-wife reside in the same house. Co-residence in a single homestead may be a new pattern associated with sedentism and the relative costs of permanent homes versus movable tents. Essential to successful cohabitation is an equitable rotation schedule. The husband and his wives must arrange a rotation schedule soon after the second marriage. Although these schedules vary, most husbands spent three to four nights with each wife.

37. Gen. 12:2 (New King James Version).

38. Gen. 15:5.

39. Gen. 16:2.

40. Gen. 16:3.

41. See Tabutin and Schoumaker, "Demography of the Arab World."

42. Syrian Arab Republic, *Maternal and Child Health Survey*.

43. Lebanon Ministry of Public Health, *Maternal and Child Health Survey*.

44. National estimates from 1993 reveal that the average duration of breastfeeding in Syria was 13.3 months (Syrian Arab Republic, *Maternal and Child Health Survey*, 10). The mean breastfeeding duration in Lebanon in 1996 was 9.1 months (Lebanon Ministry of Public Health, *Maternal and Child Health Survey*, 14).

Chapter 5. Marriage between Kin

1. Western and Arab biomedical scientists have also carved out a prominent niche for research on "inbreeding" in Middle Eastern societies. See, for example, Teebi and Farag, *Genetic Disorders among Arab Populations*. Consanguineous marriage is of interest to biodemographers and public-health researchers because mating between close biological relatives is believed to increase the risk of recessive disorders (see chapter 3).

2. To say that marriages are arranged is not to say "forced." Cross-cultural reports on arranged marriages indicate that, in most cases, men and women are consulted and rarely coerced into marriage. Meredith Small finds that out of a sample of 133 cultures, 106 (80 percent) have arranged marriages, either exclusively or in conjunction with unarranged marriages (Small, *What's Love Got to Do with It?*).

3. Bittles, "Consanguinity as a Demographic Variable" and Bittles, "Consanguineous Marriage in Contemporary Societies." Although the worldwide incidence of consanguinity is unknown, according to George P. Murdock's cross-cultural analyses, 53 percent of societies disapprove of cousin marriages, 39 percent allow for the practice, and the remaining 8 percent of societies are lacking adequate data. Of those societies that allow for the practice and for whom adequate data are provided, only 4 percent prefer parallel cousin marriage with a father's brother's child (Murdock, *Atlas of World Cultures*, 136).

4. See Joseph, "'Kissing Cousins.'"

5. Ibid.

6. Mares, "Desert Peoples," 157–58.

7. See, for instance, Rabino-Massa, Prost, and Boetsch, "Social Structure and Consanguinity."

8. See Bradburd, "Rules of the Game."

9. See Holy, *Kinship, Honour and Solidarity*; Abu-Lughod, *Veiled Sentiments*; Bourdieu, *Outline of a Theory*; Barth, "Father's Brother's Daughter Marriage,"; Khuri, "Parallel Cousin Marriage Reconsidered; and Gellner, *Muslim Society*. For a different view of patriparallel-cousin marriage as one that contributes to the extreme fission of agnatic lines and the creation of self-sufficient and self-contained minimal agnatic units, see Murphy and Kasdan, "Structure of Parallel Cousin Marriage." My own ethnographic observations suggest that agnatic fission and conflict are much more likely to result from not following normative rules of patriparallel marriage. Amity and antagonism oscillate depending on time-space contexts. The conflicting interests that existed between Bedouin and peasant at the time of the Great Syrian Revolt (1925–27) were put aside as many Bedouin tribes joined the anticolonial insurgency.

10. The women and men with whom I spoke did not mention consolidating inherited wealth in the form of livestock or land as a motivating factor in entering into consanguineous unions. It is important to remember that in land-poor Bedouin communities of the Bekaa Valley, marriages do not generally entail the transfer of great wealth. Most economic transfers at marriage are modest and tend to flow from the groom's family to the bride's family and from the groom's family to the groom and his bride (e.g., livestock inheritance). At the very least, marriage requires preparations for the wedding as well as the couple's residence at marriage. Older couples (forty and over) not fully transitioned to a sedentary lifestyle reported establishing their own tent at marriage. However, for younger married couples, new residence means either establishing a permanent independent household or a private room in the groom's family home. The wedding and household preparations are largely the groom's economic responsibility, whereas the bride's family assumes responsibility for preparing her trousseau. There is ample room for negotiating bride-price and other economic transfers. Establishing an independent household is the most important economic constraint on Bedouin family formation.

11. Abu-Lughod, *Veiled Sentiments*, 145.

12. Bourdieu, *Outline of a Theory*, 44.

13. Bradburd, "Rules of the Game," 749. The article describes how Komanchi marriage between close kin creates multiplex, layered and thicker ties between men already connected to one another by kinship and social status.

14. See Stone, "Anthropological Kinship."

15. Franklin and McKinnon, "Introduction," 13.

16. Durkheim, *Rules of the Sociological Method*, 2.

17. Giddens, *New Rules of Sociological Method*, 128–30, 69.

18. Gen. 22:2.

19. Gen. 21:12.

20. Delaney, "Cutting the Ties That Bind," 458.

21. See Firestone, "Marriageable Consanguinity."

22. Levine, "Gendered Grammar," 108.

23. Ibid., 109.

24. See Khuri, "Parallel Cousin Marriage Reconsidered"; Bittles, "When Cousins Marry"; Hussain, "Consanguineous Marriages in Pakistan."

25. The concept of power defined as "actors' attempts to get others to comply with their wants" does not necessarily imply conflict. Women's and men's interests in marriage transactions frequently overlap. See Giddens, *Central Problems in Social Theory*, 93.

26. See Barth, "Father's Brother's Daughter Marriage."

27. See Boddy, *Wombs and Alien Spirits*.

28. Recent scientific evidence suggests that consanguineous marriages may have some beneficial effects on health. There appears to be overlap in the geographic distributions of malaria, thalassemias, and other red-blood-cell conditions that protect against malaria, on the one hand, and consanguineous marriages on the other. See Denic and Nicholls, "Genetic Benefits of Consanguinity."

29. Lamphere, "Whatever Happened to Kinship Studies?," 34.

30. Giddens, *Constitution of Society*, 177. See also Giddens, *New Rules of Sociological Method*.

31. Harvey, *Condition of Postmodernity*.

32. Skolnick, *Embattled Paradise*.

33. Bedouin women and men describe a man's right to his patriparallel cousin by saying that he "clutches onto her" or "holds onto her." He has a right to her and can prevent her from marrying another even on her wedding day. This does not mean that Bedouin men are free to marry as they please. Some men also explained to me how they were obliged to marry their patriparallel cousin. For example, one married man in the company of his cousin-wife explained that although he was six years younger than his cousin and did not love her, he still had to marry her.

34. Illouz, *Consuming the Romantic Utopia*, 26.

35. Collier, *From Duty to Desire*.

36. Hirsch, *Courtship after Marriage*.

37. Adelkhah, *Being Modern in Iran*.

38. See Lefebvre, *Production of Space*.

39. For a discussion of "crossing" and "osmosis" across ethnic boundaries, see Barth, *Ethnic Groups and Boundaries*, 21.

Chapter 6. Population and Poverty

1. In the United States, population surveys indicate that, since 1990, nuclear families no longer represent the dominant family type. Estimates from 2000 indicate that there were more people living alone in America than there were married couples with children. Approximately 28.7 percent of households were comprised of married couples living without children (under age eighteen), 25.5 percent consisted of women or men living alone, 24.1 percent were married-couple families with children (under age eighteen), and the remaining 21.7 percent of households consisted of other "family and nonfamily" types (Fields and Casper, "America's Families and Living Arrangements").

2. Schneider and Schneider, *Festival of the Poor*, 191.

3. United Nations Population Fund, *State of World Population 2007*, 3.

4. See Lee, "Demographic Transition."

5. Coale and Watkins, *Decline of Fertility in Europe*.

6. Chesnais, "Comment."

7. See Easterly, *White Man's Burden*.

8. Ibid.

9. Lee, "Demographic Transition."

10. See Chesnais, "Comment."

11. United Nations Population Fund, *State of World Population 2007*, 7.

12. See Caldwell, "Globalization of Fertility Behavior." See also Chesnais, "Comment."

13. See Population Reference Bureau, *2007 World Population Data Sheet*.

14. United Nations Development Programme, *Human Development Report 2007/2008*.

15. Caldwell, "Globalization of Fertility Behavior."

16. See note 13 above.

17. Lee, "Demographic Transition."

18. Demeny and McNicoll, "Political Demography."

19. Livi-Bacci, *Concise History of World Population*, 6.

20. Ibid., 10.

21. Malthus, *Principle of Population*, 17.

22. Ibid., 34.

23. Ibid., 44.

24. For an excellent critique of Malthus's "natural law," see Harvey, *Geography of Difference*, 139–49.

25. Malthus, *Principle of Population*, 41.

26. Ibid., 208.

27. Ibid., 123.

28. Ibid., 101.

29. Ibid., 270.

30. Marx, "Malthus as an Apologist," 136; Engels, "Declaration of War," 70.

31. Malthus, *Principle of Population*, 278.

32. See Wood, "Fertility in Anthropological Populations" and Defo, "Infant and Child Survival."

33. See Lee and Feng, *One Quarter of Humanity*.

34. Another idea compatible with the Malthusian model and widely accepted is the notion that human mortality (and population growth more generally) are influenced by subsistence, particularly acute economic and environmental distress (see also chapter 7 for an examination of the role of economic forces and social class in explaining demographic transitions).

35. Lee and Feng, *One Quarter of Humanity*, 90.

36. The first major phase of Chinese population growth occurred between the eighteenth and nineteenth centuries as population increased from 150 million in 1700 to 500 million in 1900. Growing economic opportunities made available by the opening up of new rural frontier lands was a major impetus behind this growth. The second major growth phase occurred in the twentieth century as China's population grew from 580 million in 1950 to 1.2 billion in 2000 (Lee and Feng, *One Quarter of Humanity*, 115–16). This period of growth was less the result of increased economic opportunity and more a consequence of the deterioration of familial control as China was reformed into a series of communes after the revolution and at an accelerated rate during the Great Leap Forward (i.e., Mao's attempt to modernize China's economy and develop agriculture and industry so that it would rival that of the United States).

37. Macfarlane, *Savage Wars of Peace*.

38. Reid, "Low Population Growth."

39. India's population growth coincided with the expansion of British rule in India and colonial dispossession of people's resources. Up until 1600, India's population was between 100 and 125 million. The population began to rise in the nineteenth century.

The population of India was estimated at 130 million in 1845; 175 million in 1855; 194 million in 1867; and 255 million in 1871. Mies and Shiva, *Ecofeminism*, 284.

40. Henley, "From Low to High Fertility."

41. Svedberg, *Poverty and Undernutrition*.

42. Centers for Disease Control and Prevention, "How is BMI Calculated and Interpreted?"

43. Kramsch, "Old Order Amish Fertility Patterns."

44. Bedouins and Hutterites have some of the highest fertility rates ever recorded. Joseph, "Biocultural Context." See chapter 4.

45. Research shows that the relationship between BMI and mortality is U-shaped, meaning that both excessive leanness and obesity are associated with lower life expectancy. The classification put forward by WHO places Bedouin women in the Grade I overweight category (BMI 25.00 to 29.99). See Mascie-Taylor and Goto, "Body Mass Index." See also Stini, "Biology of Human Aging."

46. Historical estimates of Bekaa Bedouin fertility indicate that high fertility is of some antiquity. Bedouin women who were born in the early part of the twentieth century, between 1899 and 1933, had an estimated completed family size of 6.81. Fertility increased among women born between 1934 and 1960, who averaged around eight births (see chapter 2).

47. See Alexander, "Women, Labour and Fertility," and "Labour Expropriation and Fertility."

48. See Baba et al., "Nutritional Status of Bedouin Children."

49. Gaspard, *Political Economy of Lebanon*, 198.

50. See Federal Research Division, *Lebanon*. See also Gaspard, *Political Economy of Lebanon*.

51. Eaton and Mayer, "Social Biology."

52. Peter, *Dynamics of Hutterite Society*.

53. Marx, "Relative Surplus-Population under Capitalism," 95.

54. Ibid., 94.

Chapter 7. Class Differentiation of Demographic Regimes

1. See Coale and Watkins, *The Decline of Fertility in Europe*. See also Watkins, *From Provinces into Nations*.

2. Lesthaeghe, *Decline of Belgium Fertility*.

3. Livi-Bacci, *Century of Portuguese Fertility*.

4. Watkins, "Conclusions" and *From Provinces into Nations*.

5. Cleland and Wilson, "Demand Theories," 24.

6. Ibid., 24–25.

7. See Kertzer and Fricke, *Anthropological Demography*. For a discussion of the early rapprochement between demography and anthropology in the 1950s, see Bernardi and Hutter, "Anthropological Demography of Europe."

8. Scheper-Hughes, "Demography without Numbers," 205.

9. Fricke, "Culture Theory and Demographic Process," 256.

10. Greenhalgh, "Anthropology Theorizes Reproduction," 12.

11. See Kertzer, "Qualitative and Quantitative Approaches."

12. See, for instance, Fricke, "Culture and Causality," and Johnson-Hanks, "What Kind of Theory for Anthropological Demography?"

13. Kertzer and Hogan, *Demographic Change*.

14. "Villamaura" is a pseudonym for a town in the rural interior of Sicily. See Schneider and Schneider, *Festival of the Poor*.

15. For Italy, see Kertzer and Hogan, *Demographic Change*, 167. For Sicily, see Schneider and Schneider, *Festival of the Poor*, 114–15.

16. Kertzer and Hogan, *Demographic Change*, 179.

17. Ibid., 10.

18. See Kertzer, *Family Life in Central Italy*. See also Kertzer and Hogan, *Demographic Change*.

19. Schneider and Schneider, *Festival of the Poor*, 220–22.

20. Ibid., 220.

21. Ibid., 222.

22. Ibid., 258.

23. Ibid., 253.

24. Ibid., 259.

25. See Reay, *Microhistories*.

26. Ibid., 62, 65.

27. Ibid., 75.

28. Das Gupta, "Kinship Systems and Demographic Regimes."

29. Folmar, "Variation and Change."

30. Das Gupta, "Fertility Decline in Punjab, India," 496–97.

31. Ibid., 497.

32. Ibid.

33. Folmar, "Variation and Change," 236.

34. Ibid., 235.

35. Ibid.

36. Das Gupta, "Fertility Decline in Punjab, India," 87. The control of marriage and remarriage among landed castes/classes in India and Nepal recalls the rule of "no land, no marriage" associated with peasant peoples of northwest Europe (Macfarlane, "English Economy").

37. Watkins, *From Provinces into Nations*, 9.

38. Coale and Trussell, "Model Fertility Schedules."

39. See Wilson, Oeppen, and Pardoe, "What Is Natural Fertility?"

40. Livi-Bacci, "Social-Group Forerunners," 189.

41. Galloway, "Pre-Revolutionary France."

42. Ibid., 286. In a cross-sectional analysis, Galloway also found a minor difference of approximately one live birth between notables and laborers in Rouen, with notables having lower fertility. The proximate mechanisms of lower fertility among notables were

delayed marriage and an earlier age at last birth (Galloway, "Pre-Revolutionary France," 272).

43. Scott and Duncan, "Pre-Industrial Population," 77.

44. See note 41 above.

45. Schellekens, "Dutch Villages," 394.

46. Ibid., 396.

47. Ibid., 401.

48. Ibid., 399. The greater vulnerability of the poorer segment of the population to typhus and dysentery is attributed to differences in personal hygiene and relative over-crowding. Schellekens, "Dutch Villages," 391.

49. Scott and Duncan, "Pre-Industrial Population," 79.

50. Voland and Chasiotis, "Reproductive Fitness," 226.

51. Ibid., 227–28.

52. Ibid., 229.

53. See Sundin, "Swedish Mortality Transition."

54. See Knodel, "Demographic Transitions in German Villages" and *Demographic Behavior in the Past.*

55. Knodel, *Demographic Behavior in the Past*, 447.

56. See Fure, "Social Differences in Infant Mortality."

57. See Telford, "Chinese Genealogies" and "Fertility and Population Growth." Please note that I do not include other examples from China for reasons of incommensurability. Most of the studies on social class in China rely on lineage genealogies, a unique source for the study of China's historical demography. However, lineage genealogies usually only contain records of the patrilineal descendants of the lineage's founder. For this reason, it is not possible to determine, at least from most genealogies, how many women were at risk of conception at any given point in time, and therefore not possible to calculate fertility rates for females. The studies examined here are all based on demographic measures of women, not men. This means that the conclusions drawn from the studies examined in this chapter do not necessarily apply to men's reproductive experiences.

58. Telford, "Fertility and Population Growth," 63.

59. Ibid., 61–62.

60. See Vanlandingham and Hirschman, "Population Pressure."

61. See Henley, "Colonial Period."

62. See Vanlandingham and Hirschman, "Population Pressure," 235.

63. Ibid., 240.

64. Henley, "Colonial Period," 316.

65. Ibid., 317–18.

66. Vanlandingham and Hirschman, "Population Pressure."

67. Carr, Pan, and Bilsborrow, "Declining Fertility on the Frontier," 30.

68. Livi-Bacci, "Social-Group Forerunners."

69. Ibid., 199.

70. Das Gupta, "Fertility Decline in Punjab, India," 487–89.

71. Indonesia offers one example. While occupational data are not available, evidence

indicates that prior to colonization, Minhasan women had to be older (around the age of twenty) in order to marry. Premodern fertility control in the form of delayed marriage appears to have served as a preventive check to adjust fertility to land availability: "There are indications that scarcity of farmland on the central plateau of Minhasa, which had always been densely populated, was one reason for the traditional pattern of delayed marriage, and that the colonization of the coastland lowlands after 1850 was instrumental in bringing about the change. Another factor, it appears, was the increased availability of cash and trade goods for bridewealth payments." Henley, "Colonial Period," 313.

72. See, for instance, Notestein, "Population—the Long View" and Davis, *Human Society*. See also Cleland, "Effects."

73. An analysis of empirical trends in sixty-nine developing countries between 1960 and 1990 found that the level of social and economic development varies extensively and is a poor predictor of the timing of fertility decline (similar to the situation in Europe) (Bongaarts and Watkins, "Social Interactions," 647). However, the authors report a correlation between the rapidity or pace of fertility decline and the level of development at the onset of transition (Bongaarts and Watkins, "Social Interactions," 655). Bongaarts and Watkins measure the level of social and economic development in contemporary developing countries using individual socioeconomic variables, and a single composite measure, the human development index (HDI), which combines three socioeconomic variables: life expectancy, literacy, and the real GDP per capita. Developing countries beginning transition at low levels of development tend to experience fertility decline at a slower pace, whereas countries beginning transition after having achieved relatively high levels of development tend to undergo more rapid fertility declines. Economic forces are thus said to impact the *pace* of transition. Haines has similarly shown that the tempo of fertility decline in England and Wales was influenced by economic factors, particularly income levels. He found that fertility declined faster among higher-income groups (Haines, "Social Class"). For studies on rich-poor inequalities in health outcomes in contemporary developing countries post-transition, see Wagstaff, "Health Outcomes"; Sastry, "Developing Countries"; and Curtis, *Health and Inequality*, 84–112.

74. Galloway, Hammel, and Lee, "Fertility Decline in Prussia," 152, 156.

75. Brown and Guinnane, "Fertility Transition," 45.

76. Knodel and Van de Walle, "Lessons from the Past," 398.

77. Ibid., 399.

78. Knodel, "Demographic Transitions in German Villages," 337.

79. Galloway, Hammel, and Lee, "Fertility Decline in Prussia," 136.

80. Brown and Guinnane, "Fertility Transition."

81. For potentially conflicting evidence from China and Taiwan, see Poston, "Social and Economic Development." For an example from Brazil, see Potter, Schmertmann, and Cavenaghi, "Fertility and Development." For an example from Ghana, see Klomegah, "Socioeconomic Factors Relating to Fertility."

82. See Mason, "Explaining Fertility Transitions."

83. Potter, Schmertmann, and Cavenaghi, "Fertility and Development," 751.

84. Ibid., 739.

85. Brown and Guinnane, "Fertility Transition," 41.

86. Galloway, Hammel, and Lee, "Fertility Decline in Prussia," 141.

87. See Ahl and Allen, *Hierarchy Theory*. See also Pickett, Kolasa, and Jones, *Ecological Understanding*. For an example of the use of scale in anthropological demography to explain demographic change, see Kowalewski, "Demographic Change." For an example from geography to understand health inequalities, see Curtis, *Health and Inequality*.

88. See Vogel and Theorell, "Social Welfare Models."

Chapter 8. Demography on the Nomadic Periphery

1. Bradburd, "When Nomads Settle," 36.

2. Bradburd, *Ambiguous Relations*.

3. Ibid., 94.

4. Salzman, "Is Inequality Universal?"

5. Ibid. See also Salzman, *Black Tents of Baluchistan*.

6. Irons, "Why are the Yomut Not More Stratified?"

7. Lancaster, *Rwala Bedouin Today*.

8. See note 4 above.

9. Salzman raises the question as to whether or not demographic inequalities should be considered key evidence of social inequalities (Salzman, "Toward a Balanced Approach"). I believe that they should.

10. See Stannard, *American Holocaust*.

11. See note 4 above.

12. Giddens, *Central Problems in Social Theory*, 93. See also Giddens, *New Rules of Sociological Method*.

13. See Borgerhoff Mulder, "Datoga Pastoralists of Tanzania"; Borgerhoff Mulder and Sellen, "Pastoralist Decision-Making"; Fratkin, Galvin, and Roth, *African Pastoralist Systems*; and Roth, "On Pastoralist Egalitarianism."

14. See note 4 above.

15. See note 6 above.

16. Lancaster, *Rwala Bedouin Today*.

17. Cole, *Nomads of the Nomads*.

18. Evans-Pritchard, *Sanusi of Cyrenaica*. The Nuer of the Sudan can also be described as egalitarian (Evans-Pritchard, *Nuer*).

19. Bujra, *Politics of Stratification*.

20. Abu-Lughod, *Veiled Sentiments*. Abu-Lughod does emphasize gender hierarchy, particularly Bedouin valuation of masculinity over femininity.

21. See note 6 above.

22. Barfield, "Tribe and State Relations."

23. See note 2 above.

24. Beck, *Nomad*.

25. Black-Michaud, *Sheep into Land*.

26. Salzman, "Is Inequality Universal?" 39–40.

27. Ibid., 40.

28. Cole argues that the meaning of "Bedouin" has changed over the course of the last century. "Bedouin" no longer denotes a "way of life" anchored in ecological and economic pastoralism, but increasingly refers to an identity rooted in heritage and culture (Cole, "Where Have the Bedouin Gone?"). This changing construction of social identity appears to be directly linked to peasantization.

29. Gellner, *Muslim Society*. Gellner's observation of a "weak state and a strong culture" is applicable in this context. However, "culture" is not some mysterious external force that has a "hold over the people," as Gellner assumes, but is reproduced or modified by individual actors themselves.

30. See note 2 above.

31. For a review, see Fratkin, "Pastoralism."

32. Fratkin, Roth, and Nathan, "When Nomads Settle."

33. Sellen, "Nutritional Consequence of Wealth Differentials." Borgerhoff Mulder ("Datoga Pastoralists of Tanzania") similarly found that although economic inequalities in livestock holdings among Datoga men are pronounced, these material inequalities have not generated marked health inequalities.

34. Randall, "Low Fertility in a Pastoral Population."

35. Their data suggest that a 10 percent increase in dependence on extracted resources is associated with an increase in childhood mortality of just under thirty deaths per thousand (Sellen and Mace, "A Phylogenetic Analysis," 8).

36. Ibid.

37. Pennington, "Human Population Growth," 263.

38. Ibid.

39. See Smith, "Ethnohistory and Archaeology" and Barnard, "Kalahari Revisionism."

40. Headland and Reid, "Hunter-Gatherers" and Headland, "Revisionism in Ecological Anthropology."

41. See Kelly, *Foraging Spectrum*.

42. See Keen, "Constraints" and Cashdan, "Egalitarianism among Hunters and Gatherers."

43. Kelly, *Foraging Spectrum*, 302.

44. Lee, *!Kung San*, 244.

45. See Wilmsen, *Land Filled with Flies*.

46. Ibid., 131.

47. Ibid., 132–33.

48. Ibid., 103.

49. Ibid., 192.

50. Ibid., 297–98.

51. Ibid., 308.

52. Fischer, *Historians' Fallacies*, 296.

53. See Smith, *Conquest*.

54. Huhndorf, *Going Native*. One of the most visible manifestations of "going native" in the United States lies in the capitalistic New Age movement.

55. Torgovnick, *Primitive Passions*, 17.

56. Kelly, *Foraging Spectrum*, 296–97. A hunter-gatherer mode of production requires economic effort. Romantic depictions of modern-day Ju/'hoansi as an "original affluent society" whose members seldom toiled more than twenty hours per week is incorrect. Calculations of "work time" omitted the time spent on food-processing and cooking (Hawkes and O'Connell, "Affluent Hunters?").

57. Endicott, "Gender Relations in Hunter-Gatherer Societies."

58. Howell, *Demography of the Dobe !Kung.*

59. Hill and Hurtado, *Ache Life History*, 190–91.

60. See note 58 above.

61. See Kelly, *Foraging Spectrum.*

62. Wood, Johnson, and Campbell, "Highland New Guinea," 61–63, 69.

63. Poisson distributions resemble a normal distribution but are more tightly clustered around the mean with shorter tails.

64. Wood, Johnson, and Campbell, "Highland New Guinea," 63; and Howell, *Demography of the Dobe !Kung*, 124–25.

65. Lee, *!Kung San.*

66. Hewlett, "Sexual Selection."

67. See Kaplan and Hill, "Food Sharing among Ache Foragers."

68. Gardner and Weiner, "Social Anthropology in Papua New Guinea."

69. Howell considered the distribution to be unusual, given predictions by Cavalli-Sforza, Luca, and Bodmer that parity distributions should generally fit a negative binomial distribution, which have a variance approximately twice that of the mean. Cavalli-Sforza, Luca, and Bodmer reject the possibility that women have the same constant probability of bearing children, which implies application of a Poisson distribution. Instead, they suggest that it is only with conscious family planning that variance in the number of children is likely to decrease. See Cavalli-Sforza, Luca, and Bodmer, *Genetics of Human Populations*, 311. This view is now recognized as incorrect. The variance in TFRs in natural-fertility populations is more than three times higher than that found in populations with effective fertility control. See Wood, "Fertility in Anthropological Populations."

70. Wood, Johnson, and Campbell, "Highland New Guinea," 69.

71. Ibid. See also Wood, "Fertility in Anthropological Populations."

72. Wood, "Fertility in Anthropological Populations."

73. See Pennington and Harpending, *African Pastoralist Community.*

74. See Bailey et al., "Hunting and Gathering."

75. Malthus's chief argument—that production (food) could not keep pace with reproduction (sex) in human societies, inevitably resulting in physical distress—is flawed (see chapter 6). However, because mortality differentials are more sensitive to socioeconomic inequalities (measured by class or occupation) than fertility differentials (see chapter 7), it appears that, in general, keeping children alive poses a greater challenge for caretakers than producing live births.

76. James W. Wood, pers. comm., January 2002.

77. In a sensitivity analysis of the proximate determinants of fertility in seventy nat-ural-fertility populations, Campbell and Wood show that most of the *interpopulation* variation in fertility is due to the duration of lactational infecundability and, secondly, to the age pattern of marriage (Campbell and Wood, "Fertility in Traditional Societies," 49). However, the authors caution that their analysis provides examination of the most important proximate determinants at a highly aggregated level or across all natural-fer-tility populations. Such analyses tell us little about the proximate determinants operat-ing within populations, or *intrapopulation* variation. Intrapopulation fertility differences may be due to more physiological mechanisms (sterility and rates of fetal loss) (Wood, "Fertility in Anthropological Populations"). Bongaarts also breaks down the proximate determinants into biological and behavioral factors. Behavioral factors refer to age at marriage, the duration of postpartum infecundability (due to breastfeeding and absti-nence) and the frequency of intercourse. Biological factors, on the other hand, refer to the age at onset of sterility, intrauterine mortality and the biological risk of conceptual failure. Using a mathematical model to determine whether biological or behavioral fac-tors are more important in explaining fertility variation in ten natural-fertility popula-tions, Bongaarts determines that behavioral factors are twice as important as biological factors in explaining fertility variation in developing countries, supporting the findings of Campbell and Wood (Bongaarts, "Relative Contributions," 11).

78. See note 58 above.

79. Pennington and Harpending, *African Pastoralist Community*, 103.

80. It is not entirely clear how long STDs have been prevalent in central Africa, but infertility was not as prevalent prior to European intrusion. In particular, the rubber trade imposed by the Belgians at the turn of the century created social conditions (sexual violence) that enabled the spread of venereal disease (Voas, "Subfertility and Disrup-tion"). Caldwell and Caldwell believe that infertility started to increase around 1880, when Europeans and Arabs began to have calamitous impacts on established social rela-tions within families (Caldwell and Caldwell, "Tropical Africa").

81. Pennington and Harpending, *African Pastoralist Community*, 103.

82. Early age at first birth is associated with higher subsequent age-specific fertility among the Ache, although this pattern is not significant on reservation settlements (Hill and Hurtado, *Ache Life History*, 379).

83. Out-of-wedlock childbearing is highly uncommon among the Bedouin. No cases were identified in my research.

84. In trying to account for secondary sterility, several explanations were ruled out. First, there is no evidence of deliberate fertility limitation among women. Male infertil-ity, however, could not always be ruled out. Another contributor to secondary sterility is complications in childbirth or disease, which was a likely factor among some women, particularly first wives in polygynous marriages. That is, first wives in polygynous mar-riages had lower fertility than their co-wives. Sterility and subfertility of the first wife is an important reason that men enter into polygynous marriages in the first place (see chapter 4).

85. Vayda, "Progressive Contextualization."

86. A growing body of research suggests the presence of a significant average differ-ence in fertility between agriculturalists and nonagriculturalists across human popu-lations. Sellen and Mace estimate that for every 10 percent increase in dependence on agriculture between sister cultures, there is a fertility increase of approximately 0.2 live births per woman in their sample of sixty-nine cultural groups (Sellen and Mace, "Fertil-ity and Mode of Subsistence," 885). In terms of sedentism, evidence suggests that Ache women in Paraguay may have responded to the higher nutritional inputs and/or lower labor outputs of settled life with earlier ages of menarche and first birth. Ache women on reservations with higher previous offspring-survival rates show higher current fertil-ity probabilities, which suggests that parents were able to produce more offspring and invest more in each offspring to increase health and survivorship (Hill and Hurtado, *Ache Life History*, 379). Sedentism also appears to have increased fertility among the Agta and Kutchin, in the Philippines and the Yukon, respectively (Pennington, "Hunter-Gatherer Demography"). In contrast, Pennington and Harpending dispute Richard Lee's argument that sedentism caused higher fertility among Ju/'hoansi women. There is no evidence that the age at first birth and therefore age of sexual maturity among Ju/'hoansi women decreased (and fertility increased) in response to more food or declining activ-ity levels associated with sedentariness (Pennington and Harpending, *African Pastoralist Community*, 215).

87. See Pennington, "Hunter-Gatherer Demography."

88. The gap between marriage and first birth is partly attributable to adolescent sub-fecundity. The median age at menarche or onset of luteal function is 20.9 years. The median age at first marriage is 21.2 years (Wood, Johnson, and Campbell, "Highland New Guinea," 64–65). Cultural practices surrounding marriage may also be important, as husbands and wives do not cohabit or regularly engage in intercourse for about a year.

Chapter 9. Conclusions

1. International Labour Office, *Global Employment Trends*, 13. The new threshold for extreme poverty is US$1.25 in 2005 prices.

2. Population Reference Bureau, *2008 World Population Data Sheet*, 7–9, 11.

3. Ibid., 7–9.

4. Ibid., 3.

5. Enrique Dussel argues that the birth of the modern world system and modernity itself occurred in 1492. He conceives of modernity as the outcome of European conquest, colonization, invasion, and integration of Amerindia, which gave Europe an edge over the Arab world, India, and China. According to this view, modernity is better conceptu-alized as a "center-periphery system," as opposed to an independent European experience that signals Europe's superiority. Dussel further contends that the birth of capitalism itself—which established Europe as the "center" over the periphery in a world-system—was facilitated by Europe's violent expansion and territorial conquest (*Invention of the Americas*, 11–12). According to David Harvey, a sweeping historical-geographical shift in global economic power is currently under way, as capital is no longer flowing from East

(i.e., East Asia, especially China, and South Asia, as well as Southeast Asia) to West (i.e., the United States and Europe) (*Enigma of Capital*, 109–10). Claudia von Werlhof similarly contends that "neoliberalism marks not the end of colonialism but, to the contrary, the colonization of the North" ("Globalization and Neoliberalism," 122). Von Werlhof further adds, "The nihilism of our economic system is evident. The whole world will be transformed into money—and then it will disappear" ("Globalization and Neoliberalism," 124).

6. Marx observes that the process of capital accumulation is based on repression: "It follows therefore that in proportion as capital accumulates, the situation of the worker, be his payment high or low, must grow worse . . . It makes an accumulation of misery a necessary condition, corresponding to the accumulation of wealth. Accumulation at one pole is, therefore, at the same time accumulation of misery, the torment of labour, slavery, ignorance, brutalization and moral degradation at the opposite pole, i.e., on the side of the class that produces its own product as capital" (Marx, *Capital*, 799). One class's wealth comes at the other class's expense. Accumulation leads to an increasing concentration of the means of production and of control over labor, which expands the proletariat.

7. A primary advantage of mobile foraging for groups like the Kubu of Sumatra and the Ache of Paraguay was the freedom of movement and protection it offered from slave-raiding (Layton, "Hunter-Gatherers").

8. See Ross et al., "Income Inequality."

9. See Clifford, *Predicament of Culture*.

10. Abu-Lughod, "Writing against Culture."

11. Visweswaran, "Race," 76.

12. Farmer, "On Suffering and Structural Violence," 277. See also Farmer, "An Anthropology of Structural Violence."

13. See Mamdani, *Good Muslim, Bad Muslim*.

14. See Giddens, *Constitution of Society*.

15. Dussel, *Invention of the Americas*.

16. Harvey argues that capital accumulation is increasingly operating according to the logic of "hegemony," as opposed to the logic of colonialism and imperialism, although both logics are intertwined (*Enigma of Capital*, 204–12).

Bibliography

Aaby, Peter, Jette Bukh, Gerdi Hoff, Ida Maria Lisse, and Arjon J. Smits. "Cross-Sex Transmission of Infection and Increased Mortality Due to Measles." *Reviews of Infectious Diseases* 8, no. 1 (1986): 138–43.

Abu-Lughod, Lila. *Veiled Sentiments: Honor and Poetry in a Bedouin Society*. Berkeley: University of California Press, 1999.

———. "Writing against Culture." In *Recapturing Anthropology: Working in the Present*, edited by Richard G. Fox, 137–62. Santa Fe, NM: School of American Research Press, 1991.

Adelkhah, Fariba. *Being Modern in Iran*. New York: Columbia University Press, 2000.

Ahl, Valerie, and Timothy F. H. Allen. *Hierarchy Theory: A Vision, Vocabulary, and Epistemology*. New York: Columbia University Press, 1996.

Ahmed, Leila. *Women and Gender in Islam*. New Haven: Yale University Press, 1993.

Alexander, Paul. "Labour Expropriation and Fertility: Population Growth in Nineteenth Century Java." In *Culture and Reproduction: An Anthropological Critique of Demographic Transition Theory*, edited by W. Penn Handwerker, 249–62. Boulder: Westview Press, 1986.

———. "Women, Labour and Fertility: Population Growth in Nineteenth Century Java." *Mankind* 14, no. 5 (1984): 361–71.

Al-Faour, Fadl. "Social Structure of a Bedouin Tribe in the Syria-Lebanon Region." PhD diss., London School of Economics, 1968.

Ali, Kamran A. *Planning the Family in Egypt: New Bodies, New Selves*. Austin: University of Texas Press, 2002.

Al-Jaber, Khalifa A., and Samir M. Farid. *Qatar Family Health Survey 1998: Principal Report*. Doha, Qatar: Ministry of Health, 2000.

Alnesef, Yousef, Rashed H. Al-Rashoud, and Samir M. Farid. *Kuwait Family Health Survey 1996: Principal Report*. Kuwait: Ministry of Health, 2000.

Baba, Nahla Hwalla, Khuzama Shaar, Shady Hamadeh, and Nada Adra. "Nutritional Status of Bedouin Children Aged 6–10 Years in Lebanon and Syria under Different Nomadic Pastoral Systems." *Ecology of Food and Nutrition* 32 (1994): 247–59.

Baer, Hans A., Merrill Singer, and Ida Susser. *Medical Anthropology and the World System: A Critical Perspective*. Westport, CT.: Praeger, 2003.

Bailey, Robert C., Genevieve Head, Mark Jenike, Bruce Owen, Robert Rechtman, and

Elzbieta Zechenter. "Hunting and Gathering in Tropical Rain Forest: Is It Possible?" *American Anthropologist* 91 (1989): 59–82.

Barfield, Thomas J. *The Nomadic Alternative.* Englewood Cliffs, New Jersey: Prentice Hall, 1993.

———. "Tribe and State Relations: The Inner Asian Perspective." In *Tribe and State Formation in the Middle East,* edited by Philip S. Khoury and Joseph Kostiner, 153–82. Berkeley: University of California Press, 1990.

Barnard, Alan. "Kalahari Revisionism, Vienna and the 'Indigenous Peoples' Debate." *Social Anthropology* 14, no. 1 (2006): 1–16.

Barth, Fredrik. *Ethnic Groups and Boundaries: The Social Organization of Culture Difference.* Prospect Heights, IL: Waveland Press, 1998.

———. "Father's Brother's Daughter Marriage in Kurdistan." *Southwest Journal of Anthropology* 10 (1954): 164–71.

Basu, Alaka Malwade, and Peter Aaby, eds. *The Methods and Uses of Anthropological Demography.* Oxford: Oxford University Press, 1998.

Bearman, Peri J., Thierry Bianquis, Clifford Edmund Bosworth, Emeri van Donzel, and Wolfhart Heinrichs, eds. *Encyclopaedia of Islam.* New ed. Vol. 12. Leiden: Brill Academic Publishers, 2005.

Beck, Lois. *Nomad: A Year in the Life of a Qashqa'i Tribesman in Iran.* Berkeley: University of California Press, 1991.

Benjamin, Jessica. *The Bonds of Love: Psychoanalysis, Feminism, and the Problem of Domination.* New York: Pantheon Books, 1988.

Bernardi, Laura, and Inga Hutter. "The Anthropological Demography of Europe." *Demographic Research* 17, no. 18 (2007): 541–66.

Billig, Michael. *Freudian Repression: Conversation Creating the Unconscious.* Cambridge: Cambridge University Press, 1999.

Bittles, Alan H. "Consanguinity and Its Relevance to Clinical Genetics." *Clinical Genetics* 60, no. 2 (2001): 89–98.

———. "Empirical Estimates of the Global Prevalence of Consanguineous Marriage in Contemporary Societies." paper number 0074. Stanford: Stanford University, 1998.

———. "The Role and Significance of Consanguinity as a Demographic Variable." *Population and Development Review* 20, no. 3 (1994): 561–84.

———. "When Cousins Marry: A Review of Consanguinity in the Middle East." In *Perspectives in Human Biology. Vol 1. Genes, Ethnicity, and Ageing,* edited by Lincoln H Schmitt and Leonard Freedman, 71–83. Singapore: World Scientific Publishing, 1995.

Black-Michaud, Jacob. *Sheep into Land.* Cambridge: Cambridge University Press, 1986.

Bledsoe, Caroline H. *Contingent Lives: Fertility, Time, and Aging in West Africa.* Chicago: University of Chicago Press, 2002.

Blurton Jones, Nicholas G., Lars C. Smith, James F. O'Connell, Kristen Hawkes, and C. L. Kamuzora. "Demography of the Hadza, an Increasing and High-Density Population of Savannah Foragers." *American Journal of Physical Anthropology* 89, no. 2 (1992): 159–81.

Boddy, Janice. *Wombs and Alien Spirits: Women, Men, and the Zār Cult in Northern Sudan*. Madison: University of Wisconsin Press, 1989.

Bongaarts, John. "The Relative Contributions of Biological and Behavioural Factors in Determining Natural Fertility: A Demographer's Perspective." In *Biomedical and Demographic Determinants of Reproduction*, edited by Ronald H. Gray, Henri Leridon and Alfred Spira, 9–17. Oxford: Oxford University Press, 1993.

Bongaarts, John, and Robert G. Potter. *Fertility, Biology, and Behavior: An Analysis of the Proximate Determinants*. New York: Academic, 1983.

Bongaarts, John, and Susan C. Watkins. "Social Interactions and Contemporary Fertility Transitions." *Population and Development Review* 22, no. 4 (1996): 639–82.

Borgerhoff Mulder, Monique. "Datoga Pastoralists of Tanzania." *National Geographic Research & Exploration* 7, no. 2 (1991): 166–87.

Borgerhoff Mulder, Monique, and Dan W. Sellen. "Pastoralist Decision-Making." In *African Pastoralist Systems: An Integrated Approach*, edited by Elliot M. Fratkin, Kathleen A. Galvin and Eric Abella Roth. Boulder: Lynne Rienner, 1994.

Borofsky, Robert. "The Four Subfields: Anthropologists as Mythmakers." *American Anthropologist* 104, no. 2 (2002): 463–80.

Bourdieu, Pierre. *Outline of a Theory of Practice*. Cambridge: Cambridge University Press, 1977.

Bradburd, Daniel. *Ambiguous Relations: Kin, Class, and Conflict among Komachi Pastoralists*. Washington DC: Smithsonian Institution Press, 1990.

———. "The Rules of the Game: The Practice of Marriage among the Komachi." *American Ethnologist* 11, no. 4 (1984): 738–53.

———. "When Nomads Settle: A Critical Comment on a Critical Problem." *Nomadic Peoples* 8 (1981): 35–39.

Braveman, Paula, and Eleuther Tarimo. "Social Inequalities in Health within Countries: Not Only an Issue for Affluent Nations." *Social Science and Medicine* 54 (2002): 1621–35.

Briggs, Laura. *Reproducing Empire: Race, Sex, Science and U.S. Imperialism in Puerto Rico*. Berkeley: University of California Press, 2002.

Brown, John C., and Timothy W. Guinnane. "Fertility Transition in a Rural, Catholic Population: Bavaria, 1880–1910." *Population Studies* 56, no. 1 (2002): 35–49.

Bujra, Abdulla S. *The Politics of Stratification: A Study of Political Change in a South Arabian Town*. Oxford: Clarendon Press, 1971.

Caldwell, John C. "The Globalization of Fertility Behavior." In *Global Fertility Transition*, edited by R. A. Bulatao and J. B. Casterline, 93–115. New York: Population Council, 2001.

Caldwell, John C., and Pat Caldwell. "The Demographic Evidence for the Incidence and Cause of Abnormally Low Fertility in Tropical Africa." *World Health Statistics Quarterly* 36 (1983): 2–34.

Caldwell, John C., Palli Hanumantha Reddy, and Pat Caldwell. *The Causes of Demographic Change: Experimental Research in South India*. Madison: University of Wisconsin Press, 1988.

Campbell, Kenneth L., and James W. Wood. "Fertility in Traditional Societies." In *Natural Human Fertility: Social and Biological Determinants*, edited by Peter Diggory, Malcom Potts and Sue Teper, 39–69. London: Macmillan, 1988.

Carr, David L., William K. Y. Pan, and Richard E. Bilsborrow. "Declining Fertility on the Frontier: The Ecuadorian Amazon." *Population and Environment* 28 (2006): 17–39.

Cashdan, Elizabeth A. "Egalitarianism among Hunters and Gatherers." *American Anthropologist* 82, no. 2 (1980): 116–20.

Cavalli-Sforza, Luigi Luca, and Walter Bodmer. *The Genetics of Human Populations*. San Francisco: Freeman, 1971.

Center for Research on Population and Health (CRPH). *Patterns of Household Income and Personal Wages in Two Urban Lebanese Communities*. Beirut: American University of Beirut, CRPH, 2002.

Centers for Disease Control and Prevention (CDC), "How is BMI Calculated and Interpreted?" http://cdc.gov/healthyweight/assessing/bmi/adult_bmi/index.html# interpreted (accessed January 2010).

Chamberlain, Andrew T. *Demography in Archaeology*. Cambridge: Cambridge University Press, 2006.

Chatty, Dawn. "Bedouin in Lebanon: The Transformation of a Way of Life or an Attitude?" *International Journal of Migration, Health and Social Care* 6, no. 3 (2010): 21–30.

———. "From Camel to Truck: A Study of the Pastoral Economy of the Al-Fadl and Al-Hassana in the Bekaa Valley, Lebanon." PhD diss., UCLA, 1974.

———. *From Camel to Truck: The Bedouin in the Modern World*. New York: Vantage Press, 1986.

Chesnais, Jean-Claude. "Comment: A March toward Population Recession." In *Global Fertility Transition*, edited by Rodolfo A. Bulatao and John B. Casterline, 255–81. New York: Population Council, 2001.

Cleland, John. "The Effects of Improved Survival on Ferility: A Reassessment." *Population and Development Review* 27 (2001): 60–92.

Cleland, John, and Christopher Wilson. "Demand Theories of the Fertility Transition: An Iconoclastic View." *Population Studies* 41 (1987): 5–30.

Clifford, James. *The Predicament of Culture: Twentieth-Century Ethnography, Literature and Art*. Cambridge: Harvard University Press, 1988.

Coale, Ansley J., and Paul Demeny. *Regional Model Life Tables and Stable Populations*. 2nd ed. New York: Academic Press, 1983.

Coale, Ansley J., and James T. Trussell. "Model Fertility Schedules: Variations in the Age Structure of Childbearing in Human Populations." *Population Index* 40, no. 2 (1974): 185–258.

Coale, Ansley J., and Susan C. Watkins. *The Decline of Fertility in Europe*. Princeton: Princeton University Press, 1986.

Cole, Donald P. *Nomads of the Nomads: The Al Murrah Bedouin of the Empty Quarter*. Chicago: Aldine, 1975.

———. "Where Have the Bedouin Gone?" *Anthropological Quarterly* 76, no. 2 (2003): 235–67.

Colen, Shellee. "'Like a Mother to Them': Stratified Reproduction and West Indian Childcare Workers and Employers in New York." In *Conceiving the New World Order: The Global Politics of Reproduction*, edited by Faye D. Ginsburg and Rayna Rapp, 78–102. Berkeley: University of California Press, 1995.

Collier, Jane F. *From Duty to Desire: Remaking Families in a Spanish Village*. Princeton: Princeton University Press, 1997.

Connelly, Matthew. *Fatal Mis-Conception: The Struggle to Control World Population*. Cambridge: The Belknap Press of Harvard University Press, 2008.

Counselors, National Society of Genetic. "First Cousins Face Lower Risk of Having Children with Genetic Conditions Than Is Widely Perceived. Recommendations for Consanguinity Announced by the National Society of Genetic Counselors and the University of Washington." (April 3, 2002), http://www.nsgc.org/news/cousins.cfm.

CSDH. Closing the Gap in a Generation: Health Equity through Action on the Social Determinants of Health. Final Report of the Commission on Social Determinants of Health. Geneva: World Health Organization, 2008. http://whqlibdoc.who.int/publications/2008/9789241563703_eng.pdf.

Curtis, Sarah E. *Health and Inequality: Geographical Perspectives*. London: Sage Publications, 2004.

Curtis, Sian. L., Ian D. Diamond, and John W. McDonald. "Birth Interval and Family Effects on Postneonatal Mortality in Brazil." *Demography* 30, no. 10 (1993): 33–43.

Daher, Massoud. *The Socio-Economic Changes and Civil War in Lebanon 1943–1990*. Tokyo: Institute of Developing Economies, 1992.

Das Gupta, Monica. "Fertility Decline in Punjab, India: Parallels with Historical Europe." *Population Studies* 49, no. 3 (1995): 481–500.

———. "Kinship Systems and Demographic Regimes." In *Anthropological Demography: Toward a New Synthesis*, edited by David I. Kertzer and Tom Fricke, 36–52. Chicago: University of Chicago Press, 1997.

Davis, Kingsley. *Human Society*. New York: Macmillian, 1948.

Defo, Barthelemy Kuate. "Effects of Infant Feeding Practices and Birth Spacing on Infant and Child Survival: A Reassessment from Retrospective and Prospective Data." *Journal of Biosocial Science* 29, no. 1 (1997): 303–26.

Delaney, Carol. "Cutting the Ties That Bind: The Sacrifice of Abraham and Patriarchal Kinship." In *Relative Values: Reconfiguring Kinship Studies*, edited by Sarah Franklin and Susan McKinnon, 445–62. Durham: Duke University Press, 2001.

Demeny, Paul, and Geoffrey McNicoll. "The Political Demography of the World System, 2000–2050." *Policy Research Division Working Paper* 213 (2006).

Denic, Srdjan, and M. Gary Nicholls. "Genetic Benefits of Consanguinity through Selection of Genotypes Protective against Malaria." *Human Biology* 79, no. 2 (2007): 145–58.

Division, Federal Research. *Lebanon: A Country Study*: Kessinger Publishing, LLC., 2004.

Drevenstedt, Greg L., Eileen M. Crimmins, Sarinnapha Vasunilashorn, and Caleb E. Finch. "The Rise and Fall of Excess Male Infant Mortality." *PNAS* 105, no. 13 (2008): 5016–21.

Dupré, Georges, and Pierre-Philippe Rey. "Reflections on the Pertinence of a Theory of the History of Exchange." In *The Articulation of Modes of Production: Essays from Economy and Society*, edited by H. Wolpe, 126–60. London: Routledge & Kegan Paul, 1980.

Durkheim, Emile. *The Rules of the Sociological Method*. London: The Free Press, 1964.

Dussel, Enrique D. *The Invention of the Americas: Eclipse Of "The Other" And the Myth of Modernity*. Translated by Michael D. Barber. New York: Continuum, 1995.

Early, John D., and Thomas N. Headland. *Population Dynamics of a Philippine Rain Forest People*. Gainesville: University Press of Florida, 1998.

Early, John D., and John F. Peters. *The Xilixana Yanomami of the Amazon: History, Social Structure and Population Dynamics*. Gainesville: University Press of Florida, 2000.

Easterly, William. *The White Man's Burden: Why the West's Efforts to Aid the Rest Have Done So Much Ill and So Little Good*. New York: Penguin Books, 2006.

Eaton, John W., and Arno J. Mayer. "The Social Biology of Very High Fertility among the Hutterites: The Demography of a Unique Population." *Human Biology* 25, no. 3 (1953): 206–64.

ECODIT and Lebanon Ministry of Environment/LEDO. *Lebanon State of the Environment Report*. Beirut: Republic of Lebanon Ministry of Environment, 2001.

El Kak, Faysal. "Policy Makers and Bedouin Health Provision." *International Journal of Migration, Health and Social Care* 6, no. 3 (2010): 31–35.

El-Kholy, Heba, and Nadje Al-Ali. "Inside/Out: The 'Native' and the 'Halfie' Unsettled." In *Between Field and Text: Emerging Voices in Egyptian Social Science*, edited by Seteney Shami and Linda Herrera. Cairo: American University in Cairo Press, 1999.

Eltigani, Eltigani E. "Fertility Transition in Arab Countries: A Re-Evaluation." *Journal of Population Research* 22, no. 2 (2005): 163–83.

Endicott, Karen L. "Gender Relations in Hunter-Gatherer Societies." In *The Cambridge Encyclopedia of Hunters and Gatherers*, edited by R. B. Lee and R. Daly. Cambridge: Cambridge University Press, 1999.

Engels, Friedrich. "A Declaration of War on the Proletariat." In *Marx and Engels on the Population Bomb: Selections from the Writings of Marx and Engels Dealing with the Theories of Thomas Robert Malthus*, edited by Ronald L. Meek, 70–74. 2nd ed. Berkeley: Ramparts Press, 1971.

Evans-Pritchard, Edward E. *The Nuer: A Description of the Modes of Livelihood and Political Institutions of a Nilotic People*. London: Oxford University Press, 1940.

———. *The Sanusi of Cyrenaica*. Oxford: Oxford University Press, 1949.

Fadlalla, Amal Hassan. *Embodying Honor: Fertility, Foreignness, and Regeneration in Eastern Sudan*. Edited by Stanlie James and Aili Mari Tripp, Women in Africa and the Diaspora. Madison: University of Wisconsin Press, 2007.

FAO Technical Cooperation Programme. *Lebanon: Damage and Early Recovery Needs Assessment of Agriculture, Fisheries, and Forestry*. Rome, Italy: Food and Agriculture Organization of the United Nations, November 2006.

Farmer, Paul. "An Anthropology of Structural Violence. Sidney Mintz Lecture for 2001." *Current Anthropology* 45, no. 3 (2004): 305–25.

———. "On Suffering and Structural Violence: A View from Below." In *Social Suffering*, edited by Arthur Kleinman, Veena Das and Margaret Lock, 261–83. Delhi: Oxford University Press, 1998.

Feng, Wang, James Lee, and Cameron Campbell. "Marital Fertility Control among the Qing Nobility: Implications for Two Types of Preventive Check." *Population Studies* 49, no. 3 (1995): 383–400.

Fields, Jason, and Lynne M. Casper. "America's Families and Living Arrangements: March 2000." *Current Population Reports*, P20–537. Washington DC: U.S. Census Bureau, 2001.

Fikri, Mahmoud, and Samir M. Farid. *United Arab Emirates Family Health Survey 1995: Principal Report*. Abu Dhabi: Ministry of Health, 2000.

Firestone, Reuven. "Prophethood, Marriageable Consanguinity, and Text: The Problem of Abraham and Sarah's Kinship Relationship and the Response of Jewish and Islamic Exegesis." *Jewish Quarterly Review* 83, no. 3/4 (1993): 331–47.

Fischer, David Hackett. *Historians' Fallacies: Toward a Logic of Historical Thought*. New York: HarperPerennial, 1970.

Folmar, Steven. "Variation and Change in Fertility in West Central Nepal." *Human Ecology* 20, no. 2 (1992): 225–48.

Forste, Ranata. "The Effects of Breastfeeding and Birth Spacing on Infant and Child Mortality in Bolivia." *Population Studies* 48, no. 3 (1994): 497–511.

Frank, John, Geoffrey Lomax, Patricia Baird, and Margaret Lock. "Interactive Role of Genes and the Environment." In *Healthier Societies: From Analysis to Action*, edited by Jody Heymann, Clyde Hertzman, Morris L. Barer and Robert G. Evans, 11–34. Oxford: Oxford University Press, 2006.

Franklin, Sarah, and Susan McKinnon. "Introduction." In *Relative Values: Reconfiguring Kinship Studies*, edited by S. Franklin and S. McKinnon, 1–25. Durham: Duke University Press, 2001.

Fratkin, Elliot M. "Pastoralism: Governance and Development Issues." *Annual Review of Anthropology* 26 (1997): 235–61.

Fratkin, Elliot M., Kathleen A. Galvin, and Eric Abella Roth. *African Pastoralist Systems: An Integrated Approach*. Boulder: Lynne Rienner, 1994.

Fratkin, Elliot M., Eric Abella Roth, and Martha A. Nathan. "When Nomads Settle: The Effects of Commoditization, Nutrition and Education on Rendille Pastoralists of Northern Kenya." *Current Anthropology* 40 (1999): 729–35.

Freedman, Deborah, Arland Thornton, Donald Camburn, Duane Alwin, and Linda Young-DeMarco. "The Life History Calendar: A Technique for Collecting Retrospective Data." *Sociological methodology* 18 (1988): 37–68.

Fricke, Tom. "Culture and Causality: An Anthropological Comment." *Population and Development Review* 29, no. 3 (2003): 470–79.

———. "Culture Theory and Demographic Process: Toward a Thicker Demography." In *Anthropological Demography: Toward a New Synthesis*, edited by D. Kertzer and T. Fricke, 248–77. Chicago: The University of Chicago, 1997.

———. *Himalayan Households: Tamang Demography and Domestic Processes*. New York: Columbia University Press, 1994.

Fure, Eli. "Social Differences in Infant Mortality in the Norwegian Parish Asker and Baerum 1814–1878." *Hygiea Internationalis* 3, no. 1 (2002): 177–92.

Galloway, Patrick R. "Differentials in Demographic Responses to Annual Price Variations in Pre-Revolutionary France: A Comparison of Rich and Poor Areas in Rouen, 1681 to 1787." *European Journal of Population* 2 (1986): 269–305.

Galloway, Patrick R., Eugene A. Hammel, and Ronald D. Lee. "Fertility Decline in Prussia, 1875–1910: A Pooled Cross-Section Time Series Analysis." *Population Studies* 48 (1994): 135–58.

Gardner, Donald S., and James F. Weiner. "Social Anthropology in Papua New Guinea." In *Anthropology in Papua New Guinea: Readings from the Encyclopaedia of Papua and New Guinea*, edited by Ian Hogbin, 119–33. Carlton, Vic: Melbourne University Press, 1973.

Gaspard, Toufic K. *A Political Economy of Lebanon, 1948–2002: The Limits of Laissez-Faire*. Leiden: Brill, 2004.

Gebara, Khalil. *Reconstruction Survey: The Political Economy of Corruption in Post-War Lebanon*. Beirut: Lebanese Transparency Association (LTA); London: Tiri, 2007. http://www.tri.org/sites/www.tiri.org/files/documents/files/Reconstruction%20Survey%20Lebanon.pdf

Geertz, Clifford. "On the Devastation of the Amazon." In *Life among the Anthros and Other Essays*, edited by Fred Inglis, 123–44. Princeton: Princeton University Press, 2010.

Gellner, Ernest. *Muslim Society*. Cambridge: Cambridge University Press, 1983.

Ghosh, Bimal. *Migrants' Remittances and Development: Myths, Rhetoric and Realities*. Geneva: International Organization for Migration; The Hague: The Hague Process on Refugees and Migration, 2006.

Giddens, Anthony. *Central Problems in Social Theory: Action, Structure and Contradiction in the Social Analysis*. Berkeley: University of California Press, 1979.

———. *The Constitution of Society: Outline of the Theory of Structuration*. Berkeley: University of California Press, 1984.

———. *New Rules of Sociological Method: A Positive Critique of Interpretative Sociologies*. 2nd ed. Palo Alto: Stanford University Press, 1993.

———. *The Transformation of Intimacy: Sexuality, Love and Eroticism in Modern Societies*. Cambridge: Polity Press, 1992.

Goodman, Alan H., and Thomas L. Leatherman, eds. *Building a New Biocultural Synthesis: Political-Economic Perspectives on Human Biology*. Ann Arbor: University of Michigan Press, 1999.

Greenhalgh, Susan. "Anthropology Theorizes Reproduction: Integrating Practice, Political Economic, and Feminist Perspectives." In *Situating Fertility: Anthropology and Demographic Inquiry*, edited by Susan Greenhalgh, 3–28. Cambridge: Cambridge University Press, 1995.

———. "Controlling Births and Bodies in Village China." *American Ethnologist* 21, no. 1 (1994): 3–30.

———. "Fertility as Mobility: Sinic Transitions." *Population and Development Review* 14, no. 4 (1988): 629–74.

———. "Toward a Political Economy of Fertility: Anthropological Contributions." *Population and Development Review* 16, no. 1 (1990): 85–106.

Guess, Raymond. *The Idea of a Critical Theory: Habermas and the Frankfurt School*. Cambridge: Cambridge University Press, 1981.

Habermas, Jürgen. *Between Facts and Norms*. Cambridge: MIT Press, 1996.

Haines, Michael R. "Social Class Differentials During Fertility Decline: England and Wales Revisited." *Population Studies* 43 (1989): 305–23.

Harpending, Henry, and Patricia Draper. "Estimating Parity of Parents: An Application to the History of Infertility among The !Kung of Southern Africa." *Human Biology* 62 (1990): 195–203.

Hartmann, Betsy. *Reproductive Rights and Wrongs: The Global Politics of Population Control*. Boston: South End Press, 1995.

Harvey, David. *The Condition of Postmodernity: An Inquiry into the Origins of Cultural Change*. Cambridge, MA: Blackwell, 1990.

———. *Justice, Nature and the Geography of Difference*. Oxford: Wiley-Blackwell, 1996.

———. *The Enigma of Capital: And the Crises of Capitalism*. 2nd ed. Oxford: Oxford University Press, 2011.

Hawkes, Kristen, and James F. O'Connell. "Affluent Hunters? Some Comments in the Light of the Alyawara Case." *American Anthropologist, New Series* 83, no. 3 (1981): 622–26.

Headland, Thomas N. "Revisionism in Ecological Anthropology." *Current Anthropology* 38 (1997): 605–30.

Headland, Thomas N., and Lawrence A. Reid. "Hunter-Gatherers and Their Neighbors from Prehistory to the Present." *Current Anthropology* 30, no. 1 (1989): 43–66.

Held, Colbert C., and John Thomas Cummings. *Middle East Patterns: Places, Peoples, and Politics*. 5th ed. Boulder: Westview Press, 2011.

Henley, David. "From Low to High Fertility in Sulawesi (Indonesia) During the Colonial Period: Explaining the 'First Fertility Transition.'" *Population Studies* 60, no. 3 (2006): 390–27.

Hewlett, Barry S. "Sexual Selection and Paternal Investment among Aka Pygmies." In *Human Reproductive Behaviour: A Darwinian Perspective*, edited by Laura Betzig, Monique Borgerhoff Mulder and Paul Turke, 263–76. Cambridge: Cambridge University Press, 1988.

Hill, Kenneth, and Dawn M. Upchurch. "Evidence of Gender Differences in Child Health from the Demographic and Health Surveys." *Population and Development Review* 21, no. 1 (1995): 127–51.

Hill, Kim, and A. Magdalena Hurtado. *Ache Life History: The Ecology and Demography of a Foraging People*. New York: Aldine De Gruyter, 1996.

Hirsch, Jennifer S. *A Courtship after Marriage: Sexuality and Love in Mexican Transnational Families*. Berkeley: University of California Press, 2003.

Hoagland, Sarah Lucia. "Heterosexualism and White Supremacy." *Hypatia* 22, no. 1 (2007): 166–85.

Holy, Ladislav. *Kinship, Honour and Solidarity: Cousin Marriage in the Middle East*. Manchester, UK: Manchester University Press, 1989.

hooks, bell. *Ain't I a Woman: Black Women and Feminism*. Boston: South End Press, 1981.

Howell, Nancy. *The Demography of the Dobe !Kung*. 2nd ed. New York: Aldine De Gruyter, 2000.

Huhndorf, Shari M. *Going Native: Indians in the American Cultural Imagination*. Ithaca: Cornell University Press, 2001.

Hussain, Rafat. "Community Perceptions of Reasons for Preference for Consanguineous Marriages in Pakistan." *Journal of Biosocial Science* 31 (1999): 449–61.

Illouz, Eva. *Consuming the Romantic Utopia: Love and the Cultural Contradictions of Capitalism*. Berkeley: University of California Press, 1997.

Inhorn, Marcia C. *Local Babies, Global Science: Gender, Religion, and in Vitro Fertilization in Egypt*. New York: Routledge, 2003.

Inhorn, Marcia C., and Carolyn Fisher Sargent. "Introduction to Medical Anthropology in the Muslim World. Special Issue: Medical Anthropology in the Muslim World. Ethnographic Reflections on Reproductive and Child Health." *Medical Anthropology* 20, no. 1 (2006): 1–11.

International Labour Office (ILO). *Global Employment Trends: January 2009*. Geneva: ILO, 2009. http://www.ilo.org/wcmsp5/groups/public/@dgreports/@dcomm/documents/publication/wcms_101461.pdf.

Irons, William. "Why Are the Yomut Not More Stratified?" In *Pastoralists at the Periphery: Herders in a Capitalist World*, edited by Claudia Chang and Harold A. Koster, 175–96. Tuscon: The University of Arizona Press, 1994.

Issawi, Charles. *The Economic History of the Middle East 1800–1914*. Chicago: The University of Chicago Press, 1966.

Johnson-Hanks, Jennifer. *Uncertain Honor: Modern Motherhood in an African Crisis*. Chicago: University of Chicago Press, 2006a.

———. "On the Politics and Practice of Muslim Fertility. Special Issue: Medical Anthropology in the Muslim World. Ethnographic Reflections on Reproductive and Child Health." *Medical Anthropology Quarterly* 20, no. 1 (2006b): 12–30.

———. "What Kind of Theory for Anthropological Demography?" *Demographic Research* 16, no. 1 (2007): 1–26.

Jordan. Department of Statistics (DOS) and Macro International Inc. (MI). *Jordan Population and Family Health Survey 1997*. Calverton, MD: DOS/MI, 1998.

Joseph, Suzanne E. "The Biocultural Context of Very High Fertility among the Bekaa Bedouin." *American Anthropologist* 106, no. 1 (2004): 140–44.

———. "Globalization, Demography and Nutrition: A Bekaa Bedouin Case Study." In *Globalization, Health and Environment: An Integrated Perspective*, edited by G. Guest, 201–16. Lanham, MD: AltaMira Press, 2005.

———. "'Kissing Cousins': Consanguineous Marriage and Early Mortality in a Reproductive Isolate." *Current Anthropology* 48, no. 5 (2007): 756–64.

Kanaaneh, Rhoda Ann. *Birthing the Nation: Strategies of Palestinian Women in Israel*. Berkeley: University of California Press, 2002.

Kaplan, Hillard, and Kim Hill. "Food Sharing among Ache Foragers: Test of Explanatory Hypotheses." *Current Anthropology* 26 (1985): 223–45.

Keen, Ian. "Constraints on the Development of Enduring Inequalities in Late Holocene Australia." *Current Anthropology* 47, no. 1 (2006): 7–38.

Kelly, Robert L. *The Foraging Spectrum: Diversity in Hunter-Gatherer Lifeways*. Clinton Corners, New York: Percheron Press, 2007.

Kent, Mary M., and Carl Haub. "Global Demographic Divide." *Population Bulletin* 60, no. 4 (2005).

Kertzer, David. I. *Family Life in Central Italy, 1880–1910: Sharecropping, Wage Labor, and Coresidence*. New Brunswick: Rutgers University Press, 1984.

Kertzer, David I., and Thomas E. Fricke. *Anthropological Demography: Toward a New Synthesis*. Chicago: The University of Chicago Press, 1997.

Kertzer, David I., and Dennis P. Hogan. *Family, Political Economy, and Demographic Change: The Transformation of Life in Casalecchio, Italy, 1861–1921*. Madison: University of Wisconsin Press, 1989.

———. "Qualitative and Quantitative Approaches to Historical Demography." *Population and Development Review* 23, no. 4 (1997): 839–46.

Khawaja, Marwan, Jesse Dawns, Sonya Meyerson-Knox, and Rouham Yamout. "Disparities in Child Health in the Arab Region During the 1990s." *International Journal for Equity in Health* 7, no. 24 (2008), http://www.equityhealthj.com/content/7/1/24.

Khoja, Tawfik A., and Samir M. Farid. *Saudi Arabia Family Health Survey 1996: Principal Report.* Riyadh: Ministry of Health, 2000.

Khuri, Fuad I. "Parallel Cousin Marriage Reconsidered: A Middle Eastern Practice That Nullifies the Effects of Marriage on the Intensity of Family Relationships." *Man* 4 (1970): 597–618.

Klomegah, Roger. "Socioeconomic Factors Relating to Fertility: A Ghanian Level Test of the Contextual Theory of Fertility." *International Review of Modern Sociology* 29, no. 1 (1999): 17–33.

Knodel, John. *Demographic Behavior in the Past: A Study of Fourteen German Village Populations in the Eighteenth and Nineteenth Centuries.* New York: Cambridge, 1988.

———. "Demographic Transitions in German Villages." In *The Decline of Fertility in Europe*, edited by Ansley J. Coale and Susan W. Watkins, 337–89. Princeton: Princeton University Press, 1986.

Knodel, John, and Etienne Van de Walle. "Lessons from the Past." In *The Decline of Fertility in Europe*, edited by Ansley J. Coale and Susan W. Watkins, 390–419. Princeton: Princeton University Press, 1986.

Konner, Melvin. *The Tangled Wing: Biological Constraints on the Human Spirit.* 2nd ed. New York: Henry Holt and Co. Times Books, 2002.

Kowalewski, Stephen A. "Scale and the Explanation of Demographic Change: 3,500 Years in the Valley of Oaxaca." *American Anthropologist* 105, no. 2 (2003): 313–25.

Kraft, Dina. "A Hunt for Genes That Betrayed a Desert People." *The New York Times,* March 21, 2006, F1. LexisNexis Academic database.

Kramsch, Dieter M. "The Overlooked Roots of Old Order Amish Fertility Patterns: Malthusian or Anti-Malthusian Behavior of a Traditional Agricultural Population." working paper, Department of Sociology/Anthropology, University of Massachusetts, Dartmouth, 2008.

Kreager, Philip. "Demographic Regimes as Cultural Systems." In *The State of Population Theory: Forward from Malthus*, edited by D. Coleman and R. Schofield, 131–56. Oxford: Basil Blackwell, 1986.

Kulczycki, Andrzej, and Prem C. Saxena. "The Population, Environment, and Health Nexus: An Arab World Perspective." *Research in Human Capital and Development* 12 (1998): 183–99.

Laclau, Ernesto. *Politics and Ideology in Marxist Theory.* London: New Left Books, 1977.

Laithy, Heba, Khalid Abu-Ismail, and Kamal Hamdan. "Poverty, Growth and Income Distribution in Lebanon." Country Study no. 13. Brazil: International Poverty Centre United Nations Development Program, January 2008. http://ipc-undp.org/pub/IPCCountryStudy13.pdf.

Lamphere, Louise. "Whatever Happened to Kinship Studies? Reflections of a Feminist Anthropologist." In *New Directions in Anthropological Kinship*, edited by L. Stone, 21–47. Lanham: Rowman & Littlefield Publishers, Inc, 2001.

Lancaster, William. *The Rwala Bedouin Today*. 2nd ed. Prospect Heights, Illinois: Waveland Press, 1997.

Laughlin, Joan M. "The Evolution of Modern Demography and the Debate on Sustainable Development." *Antipode* 31, no. 3 (1999): 324–33.

Layton, Robert H. "Hunter-Gatherers, Their Neighbours and the Nation State." In *Hunter-Gatherers: An Interdisciplinary Perspective*, edited by Catherine Panter-Brick, Robert H. Layton and Peter Rowley-Conwy, 292–321. Cambridge: Cambridge University Press, 2001.

"Lebanon 1996: Results from the Lebanon Maternal and Child Health Survey." *Studies in Family Planning* 32, no. 2 (2001): 175–80.

Lebanon Department of Health and Vital Statistics. *Statistical Bulletin 2007*. Beirut: Republic of Lebanon Ministry of Public Health, October 2008. http://www.moph. gov.lb/Publications/Documents/Bulletin2007/FullBulletin2007.pdf.

Lebanon Ministry of Agriculture. *Agricultural Statistics Lebanon 2005*. Beirut, Lebanon: Food and Agriculture Organization of the United Nations Project "Support to the Agricultural Census," 2007.

———. *National Action Programme to Combat Desertification*. Beirut, Lebanon: Ministry of Agriculture, June 2003.

Lebanon Ministry of Public Health. *Lebanon Maternal and Child Health Survey. Summary Report*. Beirut: Republic of Lebanon Ministry of Public Health/League of Arab States Pan Arab Project for Child Development, 1998.

Lee, James Z., and Wang Feng. *One Quarter of Humanity: Malthusian Mythologies and Chinese Realities, 1700–2000*. Cambridge: Harvard University Press, 1999.

Lee, Richard B. *The !Kung San: Men, Women, and Work in a Foraging Society*. Cambridge: Cambridge University Press, 1979.

Lee, Ronald. "The Demographic Transition: Three Centuries of Fundamental Change." *Journal of Economic Perspectives* 17, no. 4 (2003): 167–90.

Lefebvre, Henri. *The Production of Space*. Translated by Donald Nicholson-Smith. Oxford, UK: Basil Blackwell, 1991.

Lesthaeghe, Ron. *The Decline of Belgium Fertility, 1800–1970*. Princeton: Princeton University Press, 1977.

Levine, Molly M. "The Gendered Grammar of Ancient Mediterranean Hair." In *Off with Her Head!: The Denial of Women's Identity in Myth, Religion, and Culture*, edited by H. Eilberg-Schwartz and W. Doniger, 7–130. Berkeley: University of California Press, 1995.

Lindholm, Charles. "Kinship Structure and Political Authority: The Middle East and Central Asia." *Comparative Studies in Society and History* 28, no. 2 (1986): 334–55.

Little, Michael A., and Paul W. Leslie. *Turkana Herders of the Dry Savanna: Ecology and Biobehavioral Response of Nomads to an Uncertain Environment*. Oxford: Oxford University Press, 1999.

Livi-Bacci, Massimo. *A Century of Portuguese Fertility*. Princeton: Princeton University Press, 1971.

———. *A Concise History of World Population.* 2nd ed. Malden, MA: Blackwell, 2007.

———. "Social-Group Forerunners of Fertility Control in Europe." In *The Decline of Fertility in Europe*, edited by A. J. Coale and S. W. Watkins, 182–200. Princeton: Princeton University Press, 1986.

Lockwood, Matthew. *Fertility and Household Labour in Tanzania: Demography, Economy, and Society in Rufiji District, C.1870–1986.* Oxford: Clarendon Press, 1998.

Lohman, Timothy G., Alex F. Roache, and Reynaldo Martorell. *Anthropometric Standardization Reference Manual.* Champaign, IL: Human Kinetics Books, 1988.

Macey, David. *The Penguin Dictionary of Critical Theory.* London: Penguin Books, 2000.

Macfarlane, Alan. "English Economy and Society in the Thirteenth to Fifteenth Centuries." In *The Origins of English Individualism: The Family, Property and Social Transition*, 131–64. New York: Cambridge University Press, 1979.

———. *Savage Wars of Peace: England, Japan and the Malthusian Trap.* Oxford: Blackwell, 1997.

Madi, Haifa H. "Infant and Child Mortality Rates among Palestinian Refugee Populations." *The Lancet* 356 (2000): 312.

Mahmood, Saba. "Feminist Theory, Embodiment, and the Docile Agent: Some Reflections on the Egyptian Islamic Revival." *Cultural Anthropology* 16, no. 2 (2001): 202–36.

Malthus, Thomas Robert. "An Essay on the Principle of Population." *Cambridge Texts in the History of Political Thought.* Cambridge: Cambridge University Press, 1992.

Mamdani, Mahmood. *Good Muslim, Bad Muslim: America, the Cold War, and the Roots of Terror.* New York: Pantheon Books, 2004.

Mares, Michael A. "Desert Peoples." In *Encyclopedia of Deserts.* Norman: University of Oklahoma Press, 1999.

Marmot, Michael. "Achieving Health Equity: From Root Causes to Fair Outcomes." *The Lancet* 370, no. 9593 (2007): 1153–63.

Marriott, Heidi. *Determinants of Natural Fertility Differentials: A Comparative Survey of the Rural Populations of the Inner Niger Delta of Mali.* London, U.K.: The University of London, 1993.

Marx, Karl. *Capital: A Critique of Political Economy.* Translated by Ben Fowkes. Vol. 1. London: Penguin Books, 1990.

———. "Relative Surplus-Population under Capitalism." In Marx and Engels on the Population Bomb: Selections from the Writings of Marx and Engels Dealing with the Theories of Thomas Robert Malthus, edited by Ronald L. Meek, 91–116. 2nd ed. Berkeley: Ramparts Press, 1971.

———. "Malthus as an Apologist." In *Marx and Engels on the Population Bomb: Selections from the Writings of Marx and Engels Dealing with the Theories of Thomas Robert Malthus*, edited by Ronald L. Meek, 127–38. 2nd ed. Berkeley: Ramparts Press, 1971.

Mascie-Taylor, C. G. Nicholas, and Rie Goto. "Human Variation and Body Mass Index: A Review of the Universality of BMI Cut-Offs, Gender and Urban-Rural Differences, and Secular Changes." *Journal of Physical Anthropology* 26, no. 2 (2007): 109–12.

Mason, Karen. O. "Explaining Fertility Transitions." *Demography* 34–4, no. 4 (1997): 443–54.

Massad, Joseph A. *Desiring Arabs*. Chicago: The University of Chicago Press, 2007.

Maternowska, Catherine. M. *Reproducing Inequities: Poverty and the Politics of Population in Haiti*. New Brunswick: Rutgers University Press, 2006.

Mies, Maria, and Vandana Shiva. *Ecofeminism*. London: Zed Books, 1993.

Modin, Bitte. "Birth Order and Mortality: A Life-Long Follow-up of 14,200 Boys and Girls Born in Early 20th Century Sweden." *Social Science & Medicine* 54 (2002): 1051–64.

Mohanty, Chandra Talpade. "Under Western Eyes: Feminist Scholarship and Colonial Discourses." In *Third World Women and the Politics of Feminism*, edited by Anna Russo, Chandra T. Mohanty and Lourdes Torres, 51–80. Bloomington: Indiana University Press, 1991.

Murdock, George P. *Atlas of World Cultures*. Pittsburgh, PA: University of Pittsburgh Press, 1981.

Murphy, Robert F, and Leonard Kasdan. "The Structure of Parallel Cousin Marriage." *American Anthropologist* 61 (1959): 17–29.

Netting, Robert. *Balancing on an Alp: Ecological Change and Continuity in a Swiss Mountain Community*. Cambridge: Cambridge University Press, 1981.

Notestein, Frank. "Population—the Long View." In *Food for the World*, edited by Theodore W. Shultz, 37–57. Chicago: University of Chicago Press, 1945.

Observatory/EMRO, World Health Organization/Regional Health Systems. *Health System Profile--Lebanon*. Geneva: World Health Organization EMRO, 2006.

Panter-Brick, Catherine, Robert H. Layton, and Peter Rowley-Conwy. *Hunter-Gatherers: An Interdisciplinary Perspective*. Cambridge: Cambridge University Press, 2001.

Paul, James. "Orientalism Revisited: An Interview with Edward W. Said." In *Interviews with Edward W. Said*, edited by Amritjit Singh and Bruce G. Johnson, 45–58. Oxford: University Press of Mississippi, 2004.

Pennington, Renee. "Causes of Early Human Population Growth." *American Journal of Physical Anthropology* 99 (1996): 259–74.

———. "Hunter-Gatherer Demography." In *Hunter-Gatherers: An Interdisciplinary Perspective*, edited by Catherine Panter-Brick, Robert H. Layton, and Peter Rowley-Conwy, 170–204. Cambridge: Cambridge University Press, 2001.

Pennington, Renee, and Henry Harpending. *The Structure of an African Pastoralist Community: Demography, History, and Ecology of the Ngamiland Herero*. Oxford: Clarendon Press, 1993.

Peter, Karl. A. *Dynamics of Hutterite Society: An Analytical Approach*. Alberta: The University of Alberta Press, 1987.

Pickett, Steward T. A., Jurek Kolasa, and Clive G. Jones. *Ecological Understanding: The Nature of Theory and the Theory of Nature*. 2nd ed. New York: Academic Press, 2007.

Pollock, Alex. "Sharecropping in the North Jordan Valley: Social Relations of Production and Reproduction." In *The Rural Middle East: Peasant Lives and Modes of Production*, edited by Kathy Glavanis and Pandeli Glavanis, 95–121. London: Zed Books Ltd, 1989.

Population Reference Bureau (PRB). *2007 World Population Data Sheet* Washington, DC: PRB, 2007. http://www.prb.org/pdf07/07WPDS_Eng.pdf.

———. *2008 World Population Data Sheet* Washington DC: PRB, 2008. http://www.prb.org/pdf08/08WPDS_Eng.pdf.

Poston, Dudley L. Jr. "Social and Economic Development and the Fertility Transitions in Mainland China and Taiwan." *Population and Development Review* 26 (2000): 40–60.

Potter, Joseph E., Carl P. Schmertmann, and Suzana M. Cavenaghi. "Fertility and Development: Evidence from Brazil." *Demography* 39, no. 4 (2002): 739–61.

Rabino-Massa, Emma, Michel Prost, and Gilles Boetsch. "Social Structure and Consanguinity in a French Mountain Population (1550–1849)." *Human Biology* 77, no. 2 (2005): 201–12.

Randall, Sara. "Low Fertility in a Pastoral Population: Constraint or Choice?" In *Human Reproductive Decisions: Biological and Social Perspectives*, edited by R.I.M. Dunbar, 279–96. New York: St. Martin's Press, 1995.

Ratha, Dilip, and Zhimei Xu. *Migration and Remittances Factbook 2008.* Washington DC: World Bank, 2008. http://www-wds.worldbank.org/external/default/WDSContentServer/IW3P/IB/2008/03/14/000333038_20080314060040/Rendered/PDF/429130PUB0Migr101OFFICIAL0USE0ONLY1.pdf

Reay, Barry. *Microhistories: Demography, Society, and Culture in Rural England, 1800–1930.* Cambridge: Cambridge University Press, 1996.

Reid, Anthony. "Low Population Growth and Its Causes in Pre-Colonial Southeast Asia." In *Death and Disease in Southeast Asia*, edited by Norman G. Owen, 33–47. St. Lucia: University of Queensland Press, 1987.

Renne, Elisha P. "Houses, Fertility and the Nigerian Land Use Act." *Population and Development Review* 21, no. 1 (1995): 113–26.

———. *Population and Progress in a Yoruba Town*. Vancouver: University of British Columbia Press, 2003.

Rivkin-Fish, Michele R. *Women's Health in Post-Soviet Russia: The Politics of Intervention*. Bloomington: Indiana University Press, 2005.

Ross, Nancy, Michael Wolfson, George A. Kaplan, James R. Dunn, John W. Lynch, and Claudia Sanmartin. "Income Inequality as a Determinant of Health." In *Healthier Societies: From Analysis to Action*, edited by Jody Heymann, Clyde Hertzman, Morris L. Barer and Robert G. Evans, 202–36. Oxford: Oxford University Press, 2006.

Roth, Eric Abella. *Culture, Biology and Anthropological Demography*. Cambridge: Cambridge University Press, 2004.

———. "On Pastoralist Egalitarianism: Consequences of Primogeniture among the Rendille." *Current Anthropology* 41, no. 2 (2000): 269–71.

Russell, Bertrand. *Power: A New Social Analysis*. New York: Routledge, 1992.

Sahlins, Marshall D. "The Segmentary Lineage System: An Organization of Predatory Expansion." *American Anthropologist* 63, no. 2 (1961): 322–43.

Said, Edward W. *Orientalism*. New York: Vintage Books, 1994.

Saidi, Nasser H. "Economic Consequences of the War in Lebanon." Papers on Lebanon no. 3. Oxford: Centre for Lebanese Studies, September 1986.

Salzman, Philip Carl. *Black Tents of Baluchistan*. Washington DC: Smithsonian Institution Press, 2000.

———. "Is Inequality Universal?" *Current Anthropology* 40, no. 1 (1999): 31–61.

———. "Toward a Balanced Approach to the Study of Equality." *Current Anthropology* 42, no. 2 (2001): 281–84.

Sastry, Narayan. "Trends in Socioeconomic Inequalities in Mortality in Developing Countries: The Case of Child Survival in Sao Paulo, Brazil." *Demography* 41, no. 3 (2004): 443–64.

Schellekens, Jona. "Mortality and Socioeconomic Status in Two Eighteenth-Century Dutch Villages." *Population Studies* 43, no. 3 (1989): 391–404.

Scheper-Hughes, Nancy. *Death without Weeping: The Violence of Everyday Life in Brazil*. Berkeley: University of California Press, 1992.

———. "Demography without Numbers." In *Anthropological Demography: Toward a New Synthesis*, edited by David I. Kertzer and Tom Fricke, 201–22. Chicago: The University of Chicago Press, 1997.

Schneider, Jane C., and Peter T. Schneider. *Festival of the Poor: Fertility Decline & the Ideology of Class in Sicily, 1860–1980*. Tucson: The University of Arizona Press, 1996.

Scott, Susan, and Christopher J. Duncan. "Interacting Effects of Nutrition and Social Class Differentials on Fertility and Infant Mortality in a Pre-Industrial Population." *Population Studies* 54, no. 1 (2000): 71–87.

Sellen, Daniel W. "Nutritional Consequences of Wealth Differentials in East African Pastoralists: The Case of the Datoga of Northern Tanzania." *Human Ecology* 31, no. 4 (2003): 529–70.

Sellen, Daniel W., and Ruth Mace. "Fertility and Mode of Subsistence: A Phylogenetic Analysis." *Current Anthropology* 38 (1997): 878–89.

———. "A Phylogenetic Analysis of the Relationship between Sub-Adult Mortality and Mode of Subsistence." *Journal of Biosocial Science* 31, no. 1 (1999): 1–16.

Sen, Amartya. "Population: Delusion and Reality." *New York Review of Books* 41, no. 15 (1994): 62–71.

Sheridan, Thomas E. *Where the Dove Calls: The Political Ecology of a Peasant Corporate Community in Northwestern Mexico*. Tucson: The University of Arizona Press, 1988.

Skolnick, Arlene S. *Embattled Paradise: The American Family in an Age of Uncertainty*. New York: Basic Books, 1991.

Small, Meredith F. *What's Love Got to Do with It?: The Evolution of Human Mating*. New York: Anchor Books, 1995.

Smith, Andrea. *Conquest: Sexual Violence and American Indian Genocide*. Cambridge: South End Press, 2005.

Smith, Andrew B. "Ethnohistory and Archaeology of the Ju/'Hoansi Bushmen." *African Study Monographs* Suppl. 26 (2001): 15–25.

Spivak, Gayatri Chakravorty. "Can the Subaltern Speak?" In *The Post-Colonial Studies Reader*. Edited by B. Ashcroft, G. Griffiths and H. Tiffin, 28–37. New York: Routledge, 2006.

———. "Righting Wrongs." *South Atlantic Quarterly* 103, no. 2–3 (2004): 523–81.

Stannard, David E. *American Holocaust: The Conquest of the New World*. Oxford: Oxford University Press, 1993.

Stini, William A. "The Biology of Human Aging." In *Applications of Biological Anthropology to Human Affairs*, edited by C.G.N. Mascie Taylor and Gabriel Ward Lasker, 207–36. New York: Cambridge University Press, 1991.

Stone, Linda. "Introduction: Theoretical Implications of New Directions in Anthropological Kinship." In *New Directions in Anthropological Kinship*, edited by Linda Stone, 1–20. Lanham: Rowman & Littlefield Publishers, Inc, 2001.

Sundin, Jan. "Culture, Class, and Infant Mortality During the Swedish Mortality Transition, 1750–1850." *Social Science History* 19 (1995): 117–45.

Svedberg, Peter. *Poverty and Undernutrition: Theory, Measurement, and Policy*. Oxford: Oxford University Press, 2000.

Syrian Arab Republic. Central Bureau of Statistics (CBS). *Maternal and Child Health Survey in the Syrian Arab Republic. Summary Report*. Damascus: Syrian Arab Republic Office of the Prime Minister CBS/League of Arab States Pan Arab Project for Child Development, 1995.

Tabutin, Dominique, and Bruno Schoumaker. "The Demography of the Arab World and the Middle East from the 1950s to the 2000s. A Survey of Changes and a Statistical Assessment." *Population (English edition)* 60, no. 5–6 (2005): 505–616.

Tamari, Salim. "The Persistence of Sharetenancy in the Palestinian Agrarian Economy." In *The Rural Middle East: Peasant Lives and Modes of Production*, edited by Kathy Glavanis and Pandeli Glavanis, 70–94. London: Zed Books Ltd, 1989.

Teebi, Ahmad S., and Talaat I. Farag. *Genetic Disorders among Arab Populations*. New York: Oxford University Press, 1997.

Telford, Ted A. "Fertility and Population Growth in Tongcheng County, 1520–1661." In *Chinese Historical Microdemography*, edited by Stevan Harrell, 48–93. Berkeley: University of California Press, 1995.

———. "Patching the Holes in Chinese Genealogies: Mortality in the Lineage Populations of Tongcheng County, 1300–1880." *Late Imperial China* 11, no. 2 (1990): 116–37.

Thomas, Lynn M. *Politics of the Womb: Women, Reproduction, and the State in Kenya*. Berkeley: University of California Press, 2003.

Torgovnick, Marianna. *Primitive Passions: Men, Women, and the Quest for Ecstasy*. Chicago: University of Chicago Press, 1996.

United Nations Demographic Yearbook, 2000. New York: United Nations, 2002.

United Nations Development Programme (UNDP). *Human Development Report 2007/2008. Fighting Climate Change: Human Solidarity in a Divided World.* New York: UNDP, 2007. http://hdr.undp.org/en/media/HDR_20072008_EN_Complete.pdf.

United Nations Population Fund (UNFPA). *UNFPA State of World Population 2007: Unleashing the Potential of Urban Growth.* New York: UNFPA, 2007. http://www.unfpa.org/webdav/site/global/shared/documents/publications/2007/695_filename_sowp2007_eng.pdf.

Van Hollen, Cecilia. *Birth on the Threshold: Childbirth and Modernity in South India.* Berkeley: University of California Press, 2003.

Vanlandingham, Mark, and Charles Hirschman. "Population Pressure and Fertility in Pre-Transition Thailand." *Population Studies* 55, no. 3 (2001): 233–48.

Vayda, Andrew P. "Progressive Contextualization: Methods for Research in Human Ecology." *Human Ecology* 11, no. 3 (1983): 265–81.

Velud, Christian. "French Mandate Policy in the Syrian Steppe." In *The Transformation of Nomadic Society in the Arab East,* edited by Martha Mundy and Basim Musallam, 63–81. Cambridge: Cambridge University Press, 2000.

Visweswaran, Kemala. "Race and the Culture of Anthropology." *American Anthropologist* 100, no. 1 (1998): 70–83.

Voas, David. "Subfertility and Disruption in the Congo Basin." In *African Historical Demography,* edited by Christopher Fyfe and David McMaster, 777–802. Edinburgh: Centre of African Studies, University of Edinburgh, 1981.

Vogel, Joachim, and Töres Theorell. "Social Welfare Models, Labor Markets, and Health Outcomes." In *Healthier Societies: From Analysis to Action,* edited by Jody Heymann, Clyde Hertzman, Morris L. Barer, and Robert G. Evans, 267–95. Oxford: Oxford University Press, 2006.

Voland, Eckart, and Athanasios Chasiotis. "How Female Reproductive Decisions Cause Social Inequality in Male Reproductive Fitness: Evidence from Eighteenth- and Nineteenth-Century Germany." In *Human Biology and Social Inequality,* edited by Simon S. Strickland and Prakash S. Shetty, 220–38. Cambridge: Cambridge University Press, 1998.

Wagstaff, Adam. "Research on Equity, Poverty, and Health Outcomes." In *Health, Nutrition, and Population (HNP) Discussion Paper.* Washington DC: World Bank, 2000.

Watkins, Susan C. *From Provinces into Nations: Demographic Integration in Western Europe, 1870–1960.* Princeton: Princeton University Press, 1991.

———. "Conclusions." In *The Decline of Fertility in Europe,* edited by Ansley J. Coale and Susan C. Watkins, 420–49. Princeton: Princeton University Press, 1986.

Weinreb, Alexander A. "First Politics, Then Culture. Accounting for Ethnic Differences in Demographic Behavior in Kenya." *Population and Development Review* 27, no. 3 (2001): 437–67.

Werlhof, Claudia von. "Globalization and Neoliberalism: Is There an Alternative to

Plundering the Earth?" In *The Global Economic Crisis: The Great Depression of the XXI Century*, edited by Michel Chossudovksy and Andrew Gavin Marshall, 116–44. Montreal: Global Research, 2010.

"WFP Starts Distributing Food Vouchers to Syrian Refugees in Lebanon." States News Agency, June 28, 2012. LexisNexis Academic database.

Whitworth, Alison, and Rob Stephenson. "Birth Spacing, Sibling Rivalry and Child Mortality in India." *Social Science & Medicine* 55, no. 1 (2002): 2107–19.

Wilmsen, Edwin N. *Land Filled with Flies: A Political Economy of the Kalahari*. Chicago: University of Chicago Press, 1989.

Wilson, Chris, Jim Oeppen, and Mike Pardoe. "What Is Natural Fertility? The Modeling of a Concept." *Population Index* 54, no. 1 (1988): 4–20.

Winckler, Onn. *Arab Political Demography*. Vol. One: Population Growth and Natalist Policies, Sussex Studies in Demographic Developments and Socioeconomic Policies in the Middle East and North Africa. Brighton: Sussex Academic Press, 2005.

Wood, James W. *Dynamics of Human Reproduction: Biology, Biometry, Demography*. Hawthorne, New York: Aldine de Gruyter, 1994.

———. "Fertility in Anthropological Populations." *Annual Review of Anthropology* 19 (1990): 211–42.

Wood, James W., Patricia L. Johnson, and Kenneth L. Campbell. "Demographic and Endocrinological Aspects of Low Natural Fertility in Highland New Guinea." *Journal of Biosocial Science* 17 (1985): 57–79.

World Health Organization. *The World Health Report 2001-Mental Health: New Understanding, New Hope*. Geneva: World Health Organization, 2001. http://www.who.int/whr/2001/en/whr01_en.pdf.

Yount, Kathryn M. "Excess Mortality of Girls in the Middle East in the 1970s and 1980s: Patterns, Correlates, and Gaps in Research." *Population Studies* 55, no. 3 (2001): 291–308.

Index

Page numbers in *italics* refer to illustrations.

Abu-Lughod, Lila, 99–100, 198n20

Ache foragers, 165, *166*, 167, 170, 202n86

Africa, 118, 158, 162, 165, *166*, 167, 170

African infertility belt, 170

Agency: consanguineous marriage structure, meaning and, 95–109; structuralism and, 101; of Third World women, 94

Agnatic kinship, 98, 190n9

Agricultural economy, 39, 184n28; French Mandate period and, 27, 28; sedentarization and, 170, 202n86

Agropastoralists, 4, 24, 29, 129, 167

Ahmed, Leila, 73–74

Aka Pygmies, *166*, 167–68

Algeria, 54–55

Allocative resources, 86

Amish, 126

Anabaptist Hutterites, 6–7, 126, 131

Anthropological demography, 135–36; biodemography compared with, 3; critical theory and, 9; interdisciplinary collaboration in, 10, 11, 182n20

Anthropology: critical medical, 10–11; essentializing trends in, 16–17; interdisciplinary collaboration in, 10, 11, 182n20

Anti-Semitism, dialogic repression and, 68, 187n40

Arab societies: fertility in, 37; misconceptions about, 5; stereotypes of, 178. *See also* Bedouin, Bekaa Valley; Bedouin Arabs

Argumentum ad temperantiam, 163

Arranged marriage, 83, 92–93, 115, 190n2

Autonomy, in marriage, 92–93

Balanced rivalry, 69

Barakāt, Abu, 45–46

Bavaria, 149–50

Bedouin, Bekaa Valley: BMI status by age and gender, 124–25; description, 6; dialect, 44; femininity, 78; historical estimates of fertility, 33–35, *34*; identity sources for, 49–50; in Nomadic fertility distribution, *166*, *167*; political autonomy of, 158, 199n29; TCFR, 32–33, 35, *36*, 128; TPFR, 33, 35, *36*, 128, 176. *See also* Bedouin-peasant divisions; French Mandate period; Marriage; Nomadism, Bekaa Bedouin; Pastoralism; Settlement and assimilation

Bedouin Arabs: Arabic word for, 25; citizenship, 37–38, 56; reduced mobility of, 27, 31; social economy of, 5

Bedouin-peasant divisions: context for, 46; dialogic repression in, 68, 187n40; economic disparities, 71–72; exploitation, 45; in fertility, 53–54, 55; health status, 54; peasant antipathy, 42–43; tribal affiliation and, 68–71, 187n40. *See also* Class differentiation, Bedouin-peasant

Bekaa Valley: Bekaa term, 26–27; causes of death in, 68, 187n39; demographic composition of, 38; dwellings, 22; economic trend, 32; fertility rate in, 53–54; health challenges in, 54; irrigation, 27; labor force reliant on agriculture in, 39, 184n29, 184n30; personal account of time in, 20–23; population, 37, 184n19; return trip to, 21–22; size and description, 26; territory changes in, 27–28. *See also* Bedouin, Bekaa Valley; Nomadism, Bekaa Bedouin; Pastoralism

Belgium, 134

Bible. *See* Old Testament

Biocultural synthesis, 10, 11

Biodemography, 3, 11, 160

Biogenetic factors, 4, 65–66

Biology: culture and, 104; debate over role of, 9–10; kinship and, 98, 190n9; misapplication of, 11

Birth: defects, 67; live births and survivors by occupation, 63; mean live births by marriage type, 88; peasant midwifery at, 85; spacing, 66, 80, 93, 127, 186n33, 187n35

Blood, metaphysical meaning of, 108

Body mass index (BMI), 124–25, 194n45

Botswana, 159–60, 162, 168, 170

Bourdieu, Pierre, 99–100

Bradburd, Daniel, 154–55

Breastfeeding: as contraception, 91, 93; cross-nursing, 70–71; duration, 93; health benefits of, 70–71; infant mortality and, 120, 146, 177; interruption of, 127

Bride price, 97

Bride-to-be, suicide by, 115

British-India, 124, 193n39

Camping units, 24, 25

Capitalism, 111–12, 129, 174, 179–80, 202n5, 203n6

Caste differentials, 138–40

Center-periphery system, 174, 202n5

Central African Republic, 165, 166, 167

Childbearing, class tensions and, 55–56

Child health, 81, 189n28; class disparities in, 158–59, 199n33

Child mortality. See Infant and child mortality

Children: as burden, 85; child labor, 62, 82; community raising of, 84–85; companionship provided by, 82, 87; economic benefits of, 82; gender preference of parents, 81; naming of, 44–45; of patriparallel cousins, 104; stunting and dehydration in, 54

China, 123–24, 143–44, 173, 193n36, 196n57

Christian refugees, 27

Citizenship, 37–38, 56

Civilizing mission, 15, 118

Class differentiation, Bedouin-peasant, 31–32, 72; absence of tensions, 69; childbearing and, 55–56; child mortality and, 63–64; colonialism as cause of, 54–55; cultural differences and, 42–50, 185n3, 185n4; economic markings of, 50, 50–53, 51, 52. See also Egalitarianism

Class disparity, 50, 50–53, 51, 52, 142; caste and, 138–40; child health not linked to, 158, 199n33; of demographic regimes, 133, 135–36; economic and, 50, 50–53, 51, 52; in European demographic transitions, 133–38; geographic divisions and, 161; Italian fertility decline and, 136–38; land ownership basis of, 64; micro-{#}and macrodemographics and, 145–46; in Middle-East pastoralist groups, 157; in nomadic societies, 15, 154–71, 158–60, 199n33; pretransitional, 139–45, 195n42, 196n48, 196n57, 197n71; rural England fertility decline factors of, 138; sedentarization and, 158; socioeconomic differentials and, 63–64. See also Egalitarianism

CMA. See Critical medical anthropology

Coale, Ansley, 81, 133, 140

Cole, Donald, 54, 199n28

Colonialism, 14; anthropology and, 16; Arab stereotypes resulting from, 178; class division as consequence of, 54–55; feminism coalescence with, 73–77, 187n7; fertility under Dutch-Indonesian, 145; population growth during British-India, 124, 193n39; social justice convergence with, 180; sterility legacy of, 170. See also French Mandate period; Imperialism

Commodity consumption, 113–14, 115, 126; commoditization, 128, 130, 158

Completed family size, 33, 34, 35, 35, 90–91, 93, 170, 194n46

Consanguineous marriage, 6, 14, 109–16, 190n1; agency, structure and meaning, 95–109; disapproval of, 190n3; gender disparity, 98, 106, 191n25; gender-specific benefits of, 107–8; health considerations, 66–67, 108, 191n28; prevalence by occupation, 110, 110; types, 96; worldwide incidence, 190n3. See also First-cousin marriages; Patriparallel cousin marriages

Contraception, 91–93, 130, 137, 176

Cousin marriage. See Consanguineous marriage; First-cousin marriages; Kinship; Patriparallel cousin marriages

Critical medical anthropology (CMA), 10–11

Critical theory, 11–12; social justice and, 9–16

Cross-nursing, 70–71

Culture: biology and, 104; changes in dress and, 129–30; cross-cultural fertility rates, 33;

cultural imperialism, 15; fertility differentials based on, 133–35; problems with concept, 178–79; in public discourse, 8–9; racism and, 14–15; state power and, 199n29; tribal values in terms of, 68–71

Das Gupta, Monica, 138–39, 146, 195n36
Delaney, Carol, 103–4
Delta Fulbe, *167*
Demeny, Paul, 81, 119
Demographic disparities: debate over role of biological/social forces in, 9–10; Nomadic society issues of, 154–71. *See also* Class differentiation, Bedouin-peasant; Class disparity; Economic disparities; Egalitarianism; Gender disparity
Demographic divide, 120; North-South, 42, 173–74, 202n5, 203n6; as social-justice issue, 1–3
Demographic equilibrium, 120–21
Demographic regimes, 62, 186n27; class differentiation of, 133, 135–36; ideational arguments, 133–34
Demographics: Bedouin demographic structure, 62–68, *63*; Bekaa region, 38; demographic continuities, 36; heterogeneity in, 139. *See also* Microdemography
Demographic transition, 176–77; classic model, 118; in Europe, 133–38; lag time in theory of, 130–31; revisions and confirmations, 145–52; waves of, 117–19. *See also* Pretransition
Demography: dismal science designation, 122; scale in, 149–52, 157, 169–70, 172; science of, 2–3, 122; study of health and, 179–80; units of analysis in, 149, 152. *See also* Anthropological demography; Anthropology; Microdemography
De-pastoralization, 5
Development, 13, 41; fertility decline and, 197n73; HDI and, 197n73
Dialect, Bedouin, 44
Dialogic repression, 68, 187n40
Diarrhea, 189n28
Diet, traditional Bedouin, 26
Disparities. *See* Class disparity; Gender disparity; Inequalities
Divorce, 90
Draper, Patricia, 33
Dress, transformation in, 129–30

Durkheim, Emile, 100–101
Dussel, Enrique, 179, 202n5

Ecological fallacy, 152
Economic disparities: Bedouin-peasant, 71–72; child mortality not associated with, 63–64, 65; class-specific, *50*, 50–53, *51*, *52*
Economy, Bedouin, 5, 32, 56–62, *62*; consanguineous marriage concerns of, 97, 109–16; Lebanon downturn in, 130; mixed agropastoral, 129; rise of service, 38; underground, 58. *See also* Agricultural economy; Family size
Egalitarianism, 3–4, 174; class stratification and, 163–64; conclusions on, 171–72; definitions, 156–57; family size contributing to, 84; geographical-historical explanation for, 157; mortality differentials and, 155; myth argument, 159; romanticization argument on, 162–63, 200n56
Eltigani Eltigani, 37
Emigration, 40
Empirical research: basis of current body of, 5–6; critical theory support from, 11; in micro-{#} and macrodemographics, 145–52; trends analysis in developing countries, 197n73
Engels, Friedrich, 9–10, 123, 132
Essay on the Principle of Population, An (Malthus), 8
Essentializing trends, in anthropology, 16–17
Ethnographic methods, 18–19
Eugenicism, 8, 12
Europe: class differences in pretransition Western, 140–43, 195n42, 196n48; demographic transition in, 133–38; mortality decline in, 117–18
European Fertility Project, 133–34, 136, 144–46, 148–49, 152; heterogeneity masked in, 150–51
Ex-primitives, 182n30

Family size: completed, 33, *34*, 35, 90–91, 93, 170, 194n46; gender balance and, 81, 86; high fertility and, 87, 94; land ownership and, 146–47; large families, 82–87; nuclear families, 117, 192n1; preferences, 35–36, 81–82, 85–86, 94, 128; regulation of, 91–92; small families, 87–93; weighted frequencies of, 33, *34*
Family type, in US, 192n1
Farmer, Paul, 8, 10

Farming: average farm size, 52; dry, 27; tenant, 57. *See also* Peasants; Sharecropping

Feed, 29–30

Femininity, Bedouin, 78

Feminism, 94; colonialism coalescence with, 73–77, 187n7

Feng, Wang, 123–24

Fertility: age structure, 140; Arab, 37; Bedouin-peasant differentials, 53–54, 55; Bedouin well-being and, 124–32, 194n45; cross-cultural TFRs, 33; cultural basis of differentials, 133–35; fertility-mortality link, 117, 120, 146; historical increase of Bedouin, 127; measurement of, 32, 33; methodology for estimates of, 18; in Nomadic societies, 165–71, *166, 167,* 201n77, 201nn83–84, 202n86, 202n88; occupational differences for pretransition, 141, 195n42; polygyny and, *87;* proximate determinants of, 169–70, 201n77; purported dangers of uncontrolled, 1–2; sedentarization and rising, 170–71, 202n86; sexual intercourse frequency and, 92; variation explanations, 169–70, 201n77. *See also* European Fertility Project; Fertility decline; High fertility

Fertility, Bedouin: decline in, 35–36, 37; historical estimates of, 33–35, *34;* historical perspective on, 127; parity distributions, 34, *35;* TCFR, 32–33, *35, 36,* 128. *See also* Family size

Fertility decline: Bedouin, 175–76; cause for concern over, 128–29; class differentiation in Italian study, 136–38; cultural factors emphasis in studying European, 133–35; demographic transition theory and, 147; development and, 197n73; global, 117–19; in Global South, 180; heterogeneity-homogeneity arguments, 151–52; in India, 138–39; in Prussia, 147–48; settlement and sedentarization linked to, 128

Fertility-mortality link, 117, 120, 146

Fertility rates: problematic assumptions in assessments of, 13; for world regions, 37, 184n18. *See also* Total-period fertility rate

First-cousin marriages, 114–15; love-based, 112–13; matrilateral, 107; in Middle East, 96; occupational differences in, *110,* 111; percentage of consanguinity as, 96. *See also* Patriparallel cousin marriages

Fischer, David Hackett, 9

Folmar, Steven, 139

Food sharing, 64, 70, 164, 200n56

Foragers: debate over, 159–62, 199n35; fertility distribution, *167,* 167–68, 169–70, 202n86; food sharing of, 164, 200n56; gender disparities and, 164–65; infant and child mortality, 159–60, 165, 199n35; romanticization of, 162–63; traditionalist-revisionists debate on, 160

Forced marriages, 92–93, 115, 190n2

Four Point Program, 118

Fourth World, 14, 15, 182n30

France, 141, 195n42

Free Patriotic Movement, 20

French Mandate period: Bekaa territory changes during, 27–28; census of, 28; development and military control, 27; high fertility dating back to, 127, 175; peasantization starting in, 155. *See also* Colonialism; Imperialism

Frequency of family sizes, 33

Fricke, Tom, 182n20

Fure, Eli, 143

Galloway, Patrick, 147, 151–52

Ganj, *166,* 167–68, 171, 202n88

GDP. *See* Gross domestic product

Gender, 77–81; consanguineous marriage benefits and, 107–8; division of labor, 57, 58; expectations and, 77–78; hierarchy and political egalitarianism, 198n20; kinship and, 105–6; parental preferences, 81; peasantization impact on, 78; prayer and, 78–79; pretransition mortality and, 142; relations in foraging societies, 164–65; segregation, 79

Gender-balanced families, 81, 86

Gender disparity: in child health, 81, 188n19, 189n28; consanguineous marriage and, 98, 106, 191n25; among foraging societies, 164–65; infant and child mortality, 79–81, *80,* 165, 188n19, 188n25, 189n27

Genetics, 14–15, 67

Geographic disparities, 161; global, 174, 177. *See also* Demographic divide

Giddens, Anthony, 86, 101

Global fertility decline, 117–19

Global geographic disparities, 174, 177

Global North, 12–13, 42. *See also* North-South demographic divide

Global South, 2, 12–13, 118–19; demographic disparities assertion, 42; fertility decline in, 180

Glory, power distinguished from, 86

Grazing, 24, 25, 31, 58

Gross domestic product (GDP), 39, 40, 119, 197n73

Hariri, Rafiq, 20, 37–38, 41

HDI. *See* Human development index

Health: biogenetic factors in, 4, 65–66; breastfeeding benefit to, 70–71; child, 64, 67, 81, 189n28; consanguineous marriage and, 66–67, 108, 191n28; disparities, 4, 54; measures of, 124–26; Nomadic society mortality, sociality and, 154–65; study of demography and, 179–80

Herero pastoralists, 159–60, 162, 168, 170

Heterosexualism, 76–77, 188n17

High fertility, 124–28; achievement of, 87; BMI, nutrition and, 127; family size and, 87, 94; feminism on oppression and, 73–74; among foragers, 169–70, 202n86; historical perspective on, 127; Malthusian perception of, 1, 6, 9; mortality, poverty and, 132; nutritional well-being with, 126; pathologization of, 2; progressive feminist description of, 75, 94; very, 33–34, 35, 174–75

Hoagland, Sarah, 76–77, 188n17

Home ownership, 113–14; means of production by occupation, *62*

Honor, 48–49, 69–70

Hospitality, 46–47, *47*, 48, 70

Households: construction, 51; herd size data by, *52. See also* Home ownership

Howell, Nancy, 168, 200n69

Human development index (HDI), 197n73

Hutterites, 6–7, 131

ICPD. *See* International Conference on Population and Development

Identity, Bedouin, 49–50

IMF. *See* International Monetary Fund

Imperialism, 15, 75, 93–94; racial, 180

India, 124, 138–39, 146–47, 193n39, 195n36

individualistic fallacy, 152

Indonesia, 144–45, 196n71

Inequalities: class stratification in Nomadic societies, 154–71; geographic divisions in class,

161; income, 41; Salzman on, 154–55, 198n9; scale and, 171–72; theoretical approach to, 5. *See also* Bedouin-peasant divisions; Class disparity; Demographic divide; Economic disparities; Egalitarianism; Gender disparity

Infant and child mortality, 17; ascertaining cause of death, 67–68; Bedouin marginality and, 54; Bekaa-Lebanon comparison, 53; breastfeeding and, 120, 146, 177; class differences in Western Europe, 142; consanguineous marriage increasing, 66; determinants, 66–68, 186n33, 187n35; economic disparities absent in, 63–64, 65; gender disparity, 79–81, *80*, 165, 188n19, 188n25, 189n27; infant-child mortality comparison, 81, 189n26; marriage implications of declining, 112; among nomadic foragers, 159–60, 165, 199n35; in preindustrial China, 144; pretransition, 142–43, 196n48; in Saudi Arabia, 189n27; wealth associated with, 63

Infertility, 87, 88, 89, 94, 170. *See also* Sterility

Inheritance, at marriage, 156–57

Interdisciplinary collaboration, 10, 11, 182n20

Intermarriage. *See* Consanguineous marriage

International Conference on Population and Development (ICPD), 13

International Monetary Fund (IMF), 37

Interviewees, 17, 19–21, 182n37; personal memories of nomadism, 23–24

Interview methodology, 17, 18–19, 20

Involuntary constraint, 123

Iran, 154–55

Irons, William, 156–57

Israeli war, on Lebanon, 21, 39–40

Italy, 136–38

Jordan, 80–81

Ju/Hoansi foragers, 164–65, *167*, 167–68

Kalahari foragers, 160, 161–62

Kelly, Robert, 164, 200n56

Kenya, *166*

Kertzer, David, 136, 182n20

Kinship, 99–107, 109, 177–78, 191n13; agnatic, 98, 190n9; biological factors, 98, 190n9; coercive nature of practices, 101; gender and, 105–6; modification of structures of, 115; in Old Testament, 103–4; pastoralism basis of, 114

Knodel, John, 143, 148–49
Komachi pastoralists, 154–55, 191n13
!Kung. *See* Ju/Hoansi foragers
Kuwait, 80–81

Labor, 130; child, 62, 82; gendered division of,
    57; hired out, 64, 187n45; in Lebanon, 38–39,
    184n28; population, capital and, 174
Lag time, 130–31
Lake Qaraoun, 26
Land: fragmentation, 51; landlessness, 56
Land ownership, 50–52; absentee, 56; average
    farm size, 52; class exploitation based in, 64;
    current pastoralism and, 60–61; family size
    and, 146–47; household ownership and means
    of production by occupation, 62; marriage
    constraints based on, 138–39, 195n36. *See also*
    Home ownership
Large families, 82–87; bride-price expense for,
    97; economic benefits of, 82, 86; social status
    afforded by, 84
Lebanese Maronite League, 38
Lebanon: causes of death to children under five
    in, 67–68; census of 1932, 28; child health in,
    189n28; economic downturn of, 130; fertility
    rate in, 53–54; feud between Syria and, 46;
    Israeli war on, 21, 39–40; labor force, 38–39,
    184n28; overview of study on, 8; population
    distribution in districts of, 38; regional and na-
    tional trends, 37–41; religious composition of,
    40; TFR for Bedouin compared to nation, 126
Lee, James, 123–24
Leprosy, 108
Lesthaeghe, Ron, 134
Life expectancy: for Bedouin males and females,
    81; BMI, mortality and, 194n45; demographic
    transition and, 118, 119; global average in
    2000, 125–26; in Lebanon, 53, 186n13; in less
    developed countries, 125–26, 173; as measure of
    population health, 125–26; premodern, 120
Litani River, 26
Livestock, 23, 29–30, 63, 183n44; ownership, 50,
    51, 52, 53, 62, 129, 156
Livestock, Bekaa Valley, 23, 26, 183n3
Love marriages, 112–13

Malthus, Thomas Robert, 1, 4, 8; critics of, 9;
    legacy of, 120–21

Malthusian theory, 1, 4, 6, 8, 9, 10, 121–24; Mal-
    thusian trap, 7, 120–21, 126; positive checks
    concept, 123, 193n34; pretransitional fertility
    and, 200n75; principle error in, 131; sexualiza-
    tion of poverty, 55
Marginality, infant mortality and, 54
Marriage: age, 36, 83; arranged, 95, 190n2; com-
    modity consumption impact on, 113–14, 115;
    concern for women's, 98–99; forced, 92–93,
    115, 190n2; home ownership requirement for,
    113–14; infant mortality decline implica-
    tions for, 112; inheritance at, 156–57; land
    ownership and, 138–39, 195n36; live births
    by marriage type, 88; love-based, 112–13; male
    virginity and, 48–49; matrilateral, 107; to
    nonkin, 102, 103, 105, 108; partner selection,
    49; power and, 191n25; sister-exchange, 92,
    97; stability, 90; women's autonomy in, 92–93.
    See also Consanguineous marriage; Kinship;
    Patriparallel cousin marriages; Polygyny
Marx, Karl, 9–10, 12, 86, 123, 131–32, 174, 202n6
Masculine honor, 48–49
Maternal depletion syndrome, 186n33
Matrilateral marriages, 107
McNicoll, Geoffrey, 119
Means of production by occupation, household
    ownership and, 62
Measles, 68, 188n19
Meat consumption, 26
Men: physical protection role of, 83–84; virgin-
    ity at marriage, 48–49
Microdemography, 135–36; in France, 42, 141,
    195; irony in, 153; limitations of previous
    research in, 3; macrodemography comparison
    with, 145–52; methodology, 148–49
Middle East: Bedouin tribes in, 156–57, 198n20;
    class differentiation in pastoralist, 157;
    first-cousin marriage in, 96; infant and child
    mortality gender disparities, 81, 188n25
Midwifery, 85
Migration patterns, seasonal, 24–25, 26, 29;
    change in, 127, 128; for current pastoralists,
    60, 61
Military aggression, 177, 178, 203n7
Modernization, 129–30, 202n5; fertility decline
    link to, 176
Modesty, 48
Monogamy, 90

Mortality: BMI and, 194n45; class differences for pretransition, 141–44, 196n48; decline, 117–18; egalitarianism with differentials of, 155; fertility-mortality link, 117, 120, 146; high fertility and, 132; Nomadic society health, sociality and, 154–65; nutrition-mortality link, 142; pretransitional, 142–43, 169, 200n75; scale importance in fertility and, 169–70; subsistence linked to, 193n34; subsistence modes in biodemography of, 160. *See also* Fertility-mortality link; Infant and child mortality
Murdock, George P., 190n3

Naming, of children, 44–45
Nationalization Law of 1994, 37–38
National Society of Genetic Counselors, 67
Native Indians, oppression discourse and, 74
Nature and nurture, 9
Nepal, 139
New Guinea, *166*, 167–68, 171, 202n88
NGOs. *See* Nongovernmental organizations
Nomadic societies, 154–72; child health evaluations, 158–59, 199n33; fertility in, 165–71, *166, 167*, 201n77, 201nn83–84, 202n86, 202n88; in Iran, 154–55; outside Middle East, 158–60, 199n33; sociality, mortality and health in, 154–65; state power and, 177, 203n7. *See also* Foragers
Nomadism, Bekaa Bedouin: camping units, 24, 25; first-cousin marriage and, 96; French government curtailing of, 27; identity sourced in, 49–50; migration patterns, 24–25, 26, 60, *61*; personal memories of, 23–24; transition from traditional, 23–32. *See also* Pastoralism; Sedentarization
Nongovernmental organizations (NGOs), health access improved by, 54
North-South demographic divide, 42, 173–74, 202n5, 203n6
Nuclear families, 117, 192n1
Nutrition, 124–27, 129, 194n45; capitalism and, 129; nutrition-mortality link, 142

Occupation, 23, 57; consanguineous marriage prevalence by, 110, *110*; diversification, 110, 115–16; first-cousin marriage differences in, *110*, 111; household ownership and means of production by occupation, *62*; live births and

survivors by, *63*; microdemography and, 141; pretransition differences in, 141, 195n42
Oceania, 171, 184n18
Old Order Amish, 126
Old Testament, 103–4; polygyny in, 89
Oppression, of Third World women, 12, 73–77, 187n7
Orientalism, 15, 182n35
Overpopulation, social-justice and, 2

Palestinian refugees, 189n26
Paraguay, 165, *166*, 167
Parents: gender preferences for children, 81; occupations of, 30–31, *31*
Parity distributions, fertility, 34, *35*
Pastoralism: consanguineous marriage and, 110, *110*; costs associated with, 60; current practice of, 58–61, *59, 61, 62, 62*; land ownership in today's, 60–61; Middle-East class disparity and, 157; modernization and monetization of, 29–30; 1960s major change to, 28–29; percentage of Bedouin engaged in, 23; reduced mobility and, 27, 31; term, 24; wage laborer past experience in, 65, 110. *See also* Nomadic societies
Pastoralists, Bedouin: class distinctions between peasants and, 31–32; gendered division of labor among, 58; interdependence between peasants and, 25–26, 29–30; means of production and household ownership for, *62*
Pathologization, of high fertility, 2
Patriparallel cousin marriages, 95, 104, 178; agnatic kinship and, 98, 190n9; purpose of, 98; women protected in, 106. *See also* First-cousin marriage; Kinship
Patron-client relations, 45, 185n4
Peasantization, 78, 155, 199n28; peasant-pastoralist argument, 157–58
Peasants: antipathy toward Bedouins, 42–43; Bedouin exploitation by, 45; dry farming by, 27; interdependence between pastoralists and, 25–26, 29–30; midwifery and, 85; patron-client relations, 45, 185n4; religious denigration of Bedouins, 43–44, 50. *See also* Bedouin-peasant divisions; Class differentiation, Bedouin-peasant; Farming
Poisson distribution, 167, 168, 169, 200n69
Political autonomy, 158, 199n29

Political-economy framework, 10, 174

Polygyny, 87–89, 94, 170; co-residence in, 189n36; live birth data, *88*

Population: Bekaa Bedouin, 37; Bekaa Valley, 37, 184n19; China's, 123–24, 193n36; Global North-South perceptions about, 12–13; Lebanon's distribution of, 38; Orientalism and, 15, 182n35; poverty and, 6–7; religious composition of, 40; social justice and over-, 2; world percentages for least and less-developed countries, 174

Population control, 12–13

Population growth: Bedouin-peasant class divisions, 55; in China, 124, 193n36; in India, 124, 193n39; in less and more developed countries, 119–20; Marx on, 131–32; mortality and poverty not inevitable from, 132; population bomb threat, 93–94; preventive checks to, 121–22, 124. *See also* Malthusian theory

Portugal, 134

Post-transition phase, 117

Poverty, 41; high fertility and, 132; high fertility without, 131; North-South demographic divide, 173–74; population and, 6–7; sexualization of, 55

Power: glory distinguished from, 86; marriage and, 191n25; Russel on forms of, 86; state, 156, 177, 199n29, 203n7

Prayer, 78–79

Pretransition, 117, 176–77; class differences, 139–45, 195n42, 196n48, 196n57; infant and child mortality, 142–43, 196n48; mortality in, 142, 169, 200n75; Non-European, 143–45, 196n57, 196n71; Western Europe, 140–43, 195n42, 196n48

Preventive checks, 121–22, 124

Primitives: ex-, 182n30; fascination with, 163, 199n54; romanticization of, 7–8

Progressive contextualization, 170, 175

Proletarianization, 62

Prussia, 147–50

Public health focus, 11, 182n20

Punjab, India, 138–39, 195n36

Qatar, 80–81

Qur'an, 43, 113

Racism, 14–15, 179–80

Recessive-gene expression, 67

Refugees, 27, 189n26

Relatives of the heart, 46

Remittances, 40

Reproduction: misconceptions about, 2; stratified, 42; study of, 3. *See also* Fertility; High fertility

Reproductive rights, 12, 13

Research, 16–22; challenges, 16–17; ethnographic methods, 18–19; genetic, 14–15; overview, 6–8; previous women's reproduction, 3; public health focus in, 11, 182n20

Revisionists, 160

Romanticization, 7–8, 162–63, 200n56

Russell, Bertrand, 86

Said, Edward, 15–16

Salzman, Philip, 155, 156, 198n9

Satisfaction payment, 71

Saudi Arabia, 189n27

Scale, in demography, 149–52, 157, 172; Nomadic fertility and, 169–70

Schneider, Jane, 55, 137

Schneider, Peter, 55, 137

Seasonal migration. *See* Migration patterns, seasonal

Secondary sterility, 169–70, 201n84

Sedentarization: class differentiation and, 158; commoditization and, 130; consumer outlay increase with, 126; fertility decline and, 128; fertility increase and, 170–71, 202n86

Settlement and assimilation, 28–32; gender relations and, 78–79

Sexual impropriety, 48

Sexual intercourse, frequency of, 92

Sexually transmitted diseases (STDs), 169–71

Sexual revolution, 2

Sharecropping, 30, 32, 51, 136–37; commoditization and, 128; consanguineous marriage and, 110, *110*; definition and arrangement of, 57; means of production for, *62*; percentage of Bedouin engaged in, 56–57

Sicily, 137, 146

Sister-exchange marriage, 92, 97

Small families, 87–93

Social class. *See* Class disparity

Social Darwinism, 8, 12

Social economy, 5

Social forces, debate over role of, 9–10

Social inquiry patterns, 9

Sociality, Nomadic society mortality, health and, 154–65

Social justice, 1–23; colonialism convergence with, 180; critical theory and, 9–16

Social status, from large families, 84

Socioeconomic differentials: absence of, 63–64; role of, 152–53. *See also* Class disparity

Sociology, kinship and, 98

Solidere company, 41

Spivak, Gayatri, 12, 187n7

State power, 156, 177, 199n29, 203n7

STDs. *See* Sexually transmitted diseases

Sterility, 169–70, 201n84

Stratification. *See* Class disparity

Stratified reproduction, 42

Structuralism, agency and, 101

Stunting, child development, 54

Sub-Saharan Africa, 118, 173

Subsistence, mortality linked to, 193n34

Sugar-beet mills, 29

Suicide, bride-to-be, 115

Sweden, 142–43

Syria: child health in, 189n28; child mortality and gender in, 81; feud between Lebanon and, 46; Great Syrian Revolt, 190n9

Syrian Desert, 8, 24, 25, 29, 128

Syrian shepherds, 58, 158, 187n45

Tanzania, 158

Tattooing, 43, *44*, 185n3

TCFR. *See* Total-cohort fertility rate

Tenant farming, 57, *62*

TFR. *See* Total fertility rate

Thailand, 144

Theorell, Töres, 153

Theoretical approach, to inequality issues, 5

Third World: as new phrase, 118; women's agency, 94; women's oppression, 12, 73–77, 187n7

Total-cohort fertility rate (TCFR), 32–33, *36*, 128

Total fertility rate (TFR), 32; for Bedouin compared to Lebanon national, 126; cross-cultural data on, 33; global overview, 173–74; low consumption and, 126; in pretransition Rouen, 141

Total-period fertility rate (TPFR), 32–33, *36*; for Bedouin, 33, *35*, *36*, 128, 176; in Lebanon, 53–54; in less and more developed countries, 118–19

TPFR. *See* Total-period fertility rate

Traditionalists, 160

Transportation revolution, 28–29, 31

Tribal affiliation, 68–71, 103, 112, 187n40; tribal markers, 69

Trussell, James, 140

Turkey, 96

Underground economy, 58

United Nations (UN), 118

United States (US), family types as of 2000, 192n1

Veiling, 79

Vogel, Joachim, 153

Volitional vice, 123

Wage labor, 57–58, *62*, 65, 110, *110*, 127

Weight, Bedouin women, 94, 127, 194n45

West African Sahel, 158

Western dependence, on government, 76

Western Europe, pretransitional, 140–43, 195n42, 196n48

Western feminism, 73–77, 94, 187n7

White man's burden, 117

Widowhood, 90–91, 94, 170, 201n83

Withdrawal method, 91, 92

Women: agency of Third World, 94; autonomy in marriage, 92–93; BMI for Bedouin, 124–25, 127; fertility and equality assumption, 2; initiation of polygyny by, 88; protection for, 106. *See also* Marriage

Suzanne E. Joseph is a former associate professor of anthropology at the American University of Sharjah in the United Arab Emirates. She is now an independent scholar living on the west coast of Florida.

www.ingramcontent.com/pod-product-compliance
Lightning Source LLC
Chambersburg PA
CBHW020530270326
41927CB00006B/512